THE MAGIC OF STAR DIETING

by David R. Ware, M.D.

HARRY BLOODSWORTH
6381 COOLIDGE STREET
HOLLYWOOD, FL 33024

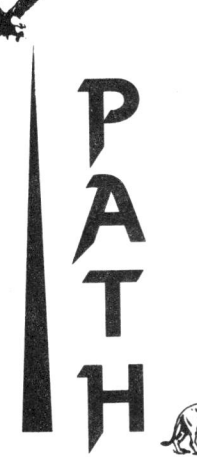

PHILOSOPHIC ASSOCIATION
OF THERAPEUTIC HOLISM

BLOOMINGTON, IN

Illustrations drawn by Tina Parker

Poetry Composed by David Ware

©July, 1987, David Ware, M.D.
All rights reserved. Published by
Philosophic Association of Therapeutic Holism, Inc.
P.O. Box 3203, Bloomington, Indiana 47402.
Library of Congress Catalog Card No. 87-72047.
ISBM 0-96184-770-0.
Manufactured in the United States of America.
No part of this book may be reproduced
without the written permission of the publisher.
Typesetting and Printing by Alexander Graphics.

second edition

*Dedicated to
Luanne & Ruth*

*the splendor of first love

casts its spell upon a lifetime*

PREFACE

This book arose out of the ancillary materials I developed for my confidential sessions with diet patients. I created a fresh way to help solve the staggering array of personal problems confounding many dieters. I became interested in dieting because I repeatedly saw a great need that was not being met elsewhere. Philosophy and empathy characterize my approach to dieting.

The goal of dieting is to consistently weigh within a narrow, desirable range- set right for yourself. However strange you may find parts of this book, I assure you that attaining good results is of utmost importance throughout. I've included only what actually works for a wide variety of people. Moreover, good *nutrition* applies from start to finish.

I assume a genuine desire to accomplish a diet resolution and I recognize the preciousness of the moment when you embark. You should only need to learn dieting once, just as you only need to learn how to drive once. You have a limited amount of starting current in the battery of your car. Most diet schemes have loose wires such that turning the ignition key, though the engine may roll over a few times, simply drains vital current- making the next attempt even less likely to succeed. Ultimately, if you try and fail often enough your battery is dead.

Basically, to get where you want to go you should do what you want to do when you're dieting. So my method respects your desires above all. If you love chocolate, steak, or chips- that's just fine. Yet since you're not the weight you want to be (though you routinely do what you want whenever you can) then your ability to steer towards your destiny must lack something in far vision (since your hands only move the way you command). You must see what you're doing to do what you want. Rather than acting impulsively - moment to moment -

perhaps you'll want to orient towards a more enduring, distant objective.

Stars evoke an ancient sense of ethereal wonder and modern intentionality. Futuristic stories vividly portray our technological reach towards the heavenly bodies. Movie stars flicker with earthly charisma. Rock stars sing to their idolizing teenage fans about pop love, fun materialism, and token rebellion.

True revolutions, however, are historically carried out by earnest adults. It is a major step from vicarious tabloid ("soap") tracking to actual enhancement of ones own level of glamor.

Successful dieting defies creeping weight increases over the years like stars seem to defy the mundane gravity weighing down human lives. Evolution towards the stars will require the wedding of science and art: **philosophy.** Philosophy can guide our civilization beyond the crucial intelligence threshold marking the transition from warring apes to *peaceful starmen.*

A magical breath of air animates our earth surface, makes the stars twinkle at night. Medical professors pollute the mental atmosphere of students with Laputanian mechanism. Thus your typical physician will admonish you to lose weight using the instructions, handouts, or diet pills provided or else ... correct advice but not truly helpful.

In despair you may turn to charlatan diet businesses that group dieters together to watch their weights go in accelerating futile cycles, spinning their wheels.

Fast food, fast money, fast computers, fast cars racing down the fast lane to instant oblivion: star wars. Some developed countries are overstuffed. "What will be thought of next?" is asked with dismay as well as appreciation. Vapid answers come zooming across the omnicient T.V. screen. The main effect of for-profit media manipulation of values is bamboozlement.

Assassins knifed Caesar to death; today a vindictive press corps can capriciously destroy a political leader via sensational insinuations and a series of malevolent barbs. The precariousness of human leadership and even life itself is self-evident. Though recent technological marvels threaten to trigger our extinction by the mere press of a button, many people sincerely seek to better their health, pleasure, and community.

Preface

Many diet books cooly indicate what to consume on a calorie, tabloid, rotational, "star" testimonial, or pseudo-scientific "potion" basis. Some authors warmly include a tincture of psychological correlation of overeating with anxiety, perhaps proselytizing a trite "way of life." This book focuses on the gateway for enhancing being as a function of intrinsic evolution with respect to unique personality and milieu: hot stuff, 'X-rated.'

The successful resolution of technologically fostered *alienation* between light and dark personal forces constitutes the main theme of this book: **romance,** the productive mating of counterpoints. The labyrinth structure of the book accords with the mental dynamics of love or dieting, quixotic states of being. The issues of love and dieting intermingle physiologically. Dieting is an *erotic* skill of pleasure management, a key element of glamor. Diet is also a potent medical force.

I eclectically use traces of Asian Martial Arts Theory, Indian Buddhism, Sufic Empiricism, Greek Philosophy, Continental Idealism, American Pragmatism, and European Existentialism along with a host of other influences (e.g. Hoosier Common Sense) to help patients succeed. Enriching the human situation is accomplished by a succession of subtle advances in what *is* rather than floundering pursuit of *ought*.

Therefore, the *modus operandi* I use to assist dieters entails confidential exchanges of ideas oriented towards optimal, intimate metaphysical change. When weight is an aberrant vital sign there exists a de novo way to improve the quality of life in both holistic and hedonistic dimensions.

Special thanks to Tina Parker for transforming my crude sketches into charming art. Sherry Cummings admirably assisted dieters in my office. I appreciate the domestic support of Gwen Ware in a venture adding much to the already considerable difficulties of a doctor's wife. The much unheralded job of homemaker-mother deserves professional respect when performed well.

I wish to express gratitude to my mother, Patricia Ware, who saved some of my off-hand notes to her and used them artistically to suggest features used in the initial design of the front cover. We all begin with mother. I also thank my father, Robert Ware, for his generous support of the pursuit of an education that contributed much to my theory of dieting.

Finally, I acknowledge the enormous intellectual stimulation of my diet patients in the genesis of this book. It was my patients who enlightened me as to the mystery, agony, and joy of learning the diet skill. A provocative process of vibrant intercourse can foster an elegant quality of living.

David R. Ware, M.D.

Full Moon
March, 1987

ABBREVIATED CONTENTS

Preface i

Part I — OVERTURE

Chapter 1	Introduction	1
Chapter 2	Resolution	6
Chapter 3	Fat	12
Chapter 4	Poison	19
Chapter 5	Exercise & Positive Pain	24
Chapter 6	Good Vision	27
Chapter 7	Caveats & Negative Pain	30
Chapter 8	Sex & Food	34
Chapter 9	Personal Time	40
Chapter 10	Civil War	43
Chapter 11	Daily Waltz	49
Chapter 12	Mentor	55

Part II — COUNTERPOINTS

Chapter 13	Dietbusters	61
13.1	Desires	62
13.2	Fears	69
13.3	Specious Reasoning	87
13.4	Intimates & Trigger Points	113
13.5	Nonintimates	123
13.6	Miscellaneous	130

Part III — FINALE

Chapter 14	Void	137
Chapter 15	Constitutional Climax	139
Chapter 16	Dividends	145
Chapter 17	Follow-Up	148
Appendix I	'Terminology' & Special Symbols	149
Appendix II	General References & Notes	158
	About the Author	163

CONTENTS

Preface, pg i

Part I   OVERTURE

Chapter 1
Introduction, pg 1
    Figure 1   Grips on Life, pg 2
    Poem 1   Eurydice, pg 5

Chapter 2
Resolution, pg 6
    Poem 2   Resolution, pg 6
    Figure 2   Outcomes, Master Graphs, pg 8
    Figure 3   Dynamic View of Aging, pg 10

Chapter 3
Fat, pg 12
    Table 1   Fat Zones of Dieting, pg 15

Chapter 4
Poison, pg 19
    Poem 3   Invitation, pg 19
    Figure 4   Body Interconversions, pg 20
    Figure 5   Fork, pg 22

Chapter 5
Exercise & Positive Pain, pg 24

Chapter 6
Good Vision, pg 27
    Table 2   Diet Constellations, pg 28

Chapter 7
   Caveats & Negative Pain, pg 30
      Table 3   Minimum Food Per Day, pg 32
      Poem 4   Warning, pg 33

Chapter 8
   Sex & Food, pg 34
      Figure 6   High Wires, pg 36
      Fragment 1 Timeless, pg 34
      Figure 7   Ideal Dieting Day, pg 38

Chapter 9
   Personal Time, pg 40

Chapter 10
   Civil War, pg 43
      Figure 8   Diet Road, pg 44
      Figure 9   Composite Dietbuster, pg 46
      Figure 10 Protean Resistances, pg 48

Chapter 11
   Daily Waltz, pg 49
      Table 4   Waltz Step Equations, pg 49
      Table 5   Final Hunger Levels, pg 53

Chapter 12
   Mentor, pg 55

          Part II   COUNTERPOINTS

Chapter 13
   Dietbusters, pg 61
   13.00   Introduction   61
             Fragment 2   Finale, pg 61
   13.10   **Desires**   62
   13.11   Scale Junky   63
   13.12   Routine Seductions   63
   13.13   Special Seductions   64

13.14	Addictions	65
13.15	Distractive Seductions	68
13.200	**Fears**	69
	Poem 5 Dark Resolution, pg 70	
13.201	Anxiety	71
	Poem 6 Waking, pg 72	
13.202	Pain	72
13.203	Intractability	74
13.204	Familial Fear	76
13.205	Jealousy	76
13.206	Sexuality	78
13.207	Highs & Lows in Feeling	80
	Poem 7 Nature's Parts, pg 81	
13.208	Protean Resistances	82
13.209	Gauntness & Fat Distribution	83
13.210	Choking	84
13.211	"Is that all?"	86
	Fragment 3 Death, pg 86	
13.300	**'Specious Reasoning'**	87
13.301	"I'm too busy!" & "I forgot."	88
13.302	"It's impossible!"	89
13.303	'Pretender'	90
13.304	Morning Faster	91
13.305	"If her then why not me too?"	92
13.306	Abortive Onset	93
13.307	"It's not fair!"	94
13.308	"I hate to be hungry!" & "I'm starving!"	95
13.309	"I have no will power."	96
13.310	Spinning Wheels	96
13.311	Tangential Approach	97
13.312	'License to Eat'	99
13.313	Calorie Counting & Hot Numbers	99
13.314	Premature Reward & Pay-as-you-go?	101
	Figure 11 Hull Holes to Hell, pg 102	
13.315	"Just a Little" Sin & Noble Cheating	101
	Figure 12 Victory or Defeat?, pg 104	
13.316	Glib "No, no" & The Big "X"	105
13.317	"I don't feel like it!" & Sour Grapes	106

13.318	Astonishing Failure	107
	Poem 8 Universal Education, pg 107	
	Poem 9 Elusive Nature, pg 108	
13.319	Fatty Martyrdom	109
13.320	"The pills don't work!"	110
13.321	Wrong Goals	110
13.322	End Point Mirage	111
13.323	Runaways	112
13.40	**Intimates & Trigger Points**	113
13.41	Real Loss	114
	Poem 10 Meeting in Dreams, pg 114	
	Poem 11 Towards New Moon, pg 115	
13.42	Imagined Loss	115
	Poem 12 Infertility, pg 116	
13.43	Ambush Weights	117
13.44	Spouse	118
13.45	Friends?	119
13.46	Children & Dependents	120
13.47	'Semi-intimate' Society	120
13.50	**Nonintimates**	123
13.51	Unstructed Time	123
13.52	Evening Binge	124
13.53	Boss & Co-workers	125
	Poem 13 Job Hunting, pg 125	
13.54	'Malmentor'	126
13.55	Commercial Gauntlets	127
13.56	Evanescent Concentration	129
13.60	**Miscellaneous**	130
13.61	Great Projects	131
13.62	Near Miss	131
13.63	Hit	132
13.64	Delicacy	132
	Poem 14 Towards Loving, pg 133	

Part III FINALE

Chapter 14
Void, pg 137

Chapter 15
Constitutional Climax, pg 139
    Figure 13 The High Tortoise, Animal of Inspiration,
               Diet Champion, pg 141
    Poem 15 Warrior's Heart, pg 144

Chapter 16
Dividends, pg 145
    Poem 16 Exotic Culmination, pg 145
    Poem 17 Ode to a Once Fat Teacher, pg 146
    Fragment 4 Dedication, pg 147

Chapter 17
Follow-up, pg 148

Appendix I   **'Terminology' & Special Symbols, pg 149**
               note: KISMET (fortune) symbols
               herein defined alphabetically

Appendix II **General References & Notes, pg 158**
               note: poetic license personified

About the Author, pg 163

List of Illustrations

Figure 1	Grips on Life	2
Figure 2	Five Typical Resolution Outcomes, Master Graphs	8
Figure 3	Dynamic View of Aging	10
Figure 4	Lightning Interconversions of Fattening Foods in the Body and the Association of Excess Salt with Water Rention	20
Figure 5	Fork	22
Figure 6	High Wires	36
Figure 7	Sample Ideal Dieting Day	38
Figure 8	Diet Road	44
Figure 9	Composite Dietbuster	46
Figure 10	Protean Resistances	48
Figure 11	Hull Holes to Hell	102
Figure 12	Defeat or Victory?	104
Figure 13	The High Tortoise, Animal of Inspiration, Diet Champion	141

List of Tables

Table 1	Selected Diet Revolution Features at Different Fat Zones	15
Table 2	Diet Constellations to Steer By	28
Table 3	Nonideal Approximate Minimum Consumption Each Day to Maintain Health Dieting	32
Table 4	Waltz Step Equations	49
Table 5	Final Hunger Level Quantitation	53

List of Poetry

Poem 1	Eurydice	5
Poem 2	Resolution	6
Poem 3	Invitation	19
Poem 4	Warning	33
Poem 5	Dark Resolution	70
Poem 6	Waking	72
Poem 7	Nature's Parts	81
Poem 8	Universal Education	108
Poem 9	Elusive Nature	108
Poem 10	Meeting in Dreams	114
Poem 11	Towards New Moon	115
Poem 12	Infertility	116
Poem 13	Job Hunting	125
Poem 14	Towards Loving	133
Poem 15	Warrior's Heart	144
Poem 16	Exotic Culmination	145
Poem 17	Ode to a Once Fat Teacher	146

List of Fragments

Fragment 1	Timeless	34
Fragment 2	Finale	61
Fragment 3	Death	86
Fragment 4	Dedication	147

Part I
OVERTURE

CHAPTER 1
INTRODUCTION

Imagine you're a *naked* woman swinging through the tall jungle trees of life. You notice the onset of some troubling slippage: winded so much more easily, and the men don't turn their heads to watch you like they once did (fig. 1.1). You even begin to consider that you might actually fall to the ground someday—morbidity.

Figure 1 illustrates how your current four-fingered "α grip" now emphasizes the social skills finger. You've forgotten the unique way you sought dramatic new psychomotor skills like walking, steering, dancing, or sex. You've yet to rediscover that you still have a thumb in an infantile sense. You used to suck your thumb as an infant (and you still retain a keen interest in putting things in your mouth for pleasure). This thumb represents a satisfying, independent capacity for evolution beyond social expectations ("α grip" is standard in your tribe).

So you pause on a remote limb and look at your hand curiously for the first time as an adult (fig. 1.2). You proudly see a unique fingerprint of femininity and realize there's a life line of destiny yet to be pursued (fig. 1.3). You're sure your hands do exactly what you command; no evil spirits direct your hand movements in eating nor anything else.

As your hands wander over your naked body you feel disgusting rolls of fat that weren't there when you mated for the first time (you've since been "so busy" doing for other people, 13.301); it's this disgusting fat that really taxes your grip on life—pulls you down.

You consider how, for a start, to get rid of this unwanted fat and recall that group of chattering semi-professional "diet talkers" that seem so smart about dieting when they meet together. But you discard the idea of joining when you note that virtually

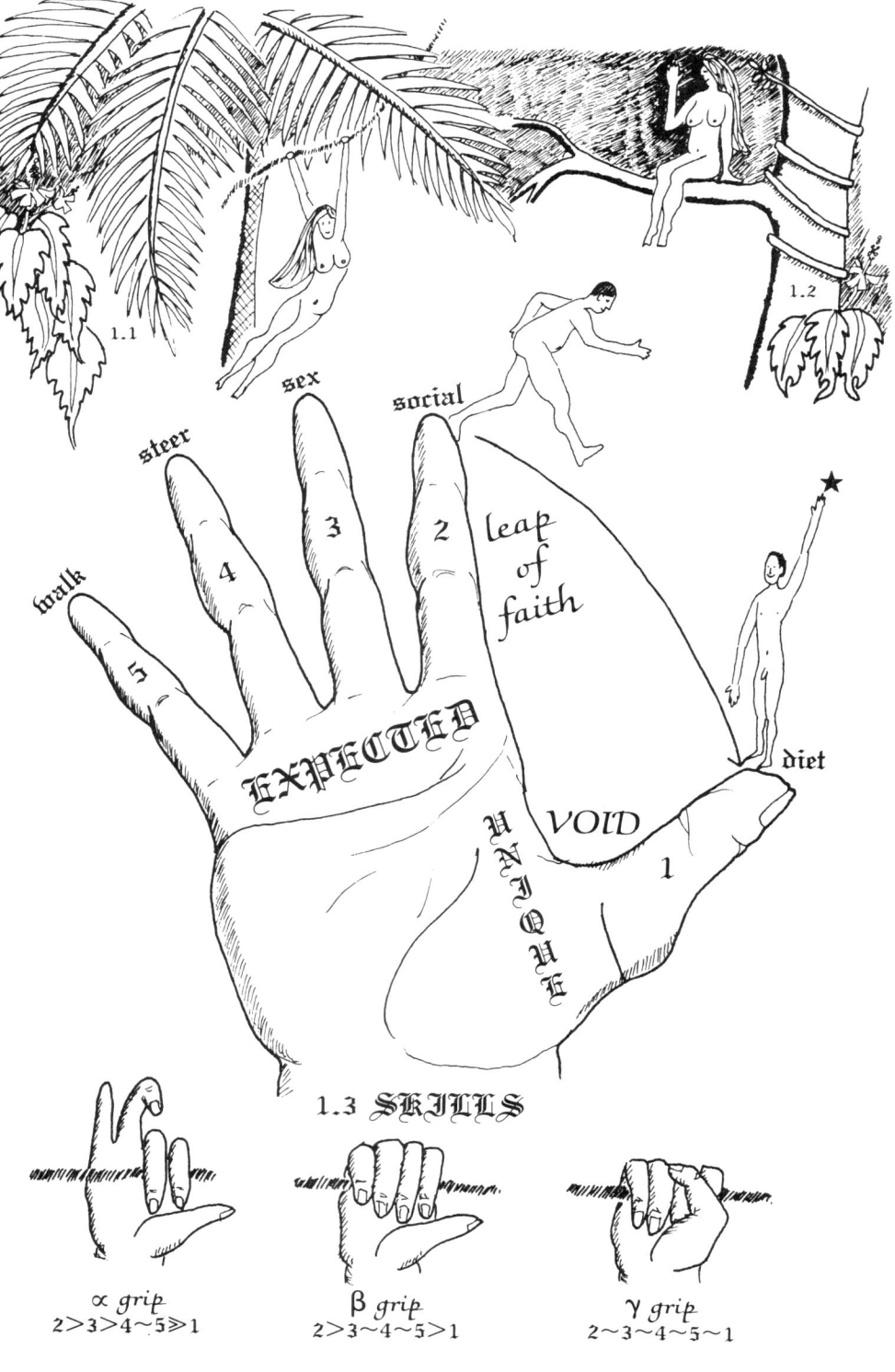

Figure 1. **Grips on Life**

all of them are quite fat, always. The average level of fatness doesn't change for the group as a whole: despite all the money spent and whooping.

Of course, you also consider good nutrition a necessary part of dieting and so rightly decide to pay particular attention to your local *witch doctor* (fig. 8). He speaks strangely but is both knowledgeable and caring (e.g. about how to learn "γ grip"). . .

By this illustration we begin to acquire the discrete **diet skill** together. We distinguish 'true dieting' from 'pretender' dieting—the latter done for a variety of reasons (13.303). When aging amplifies the downward pull of gravity on the body, then the "α grip" proves distinctly inferior to the "γ grip." The thumb, though somewhat in opposition to the other fingers (routine social forces, 13.40, 13.50), can greatly improve the quality of grip on life by working in concert with the "social skills." Transitional "β grip" involves rekindling your childhood willingness to acquire a gamut of initially awkward psychomotor skills—such as doing a 'diet diary' or slapping one hand with the other when reaching for sweets.

Further imagine a strange "diet bicycle" must be successfully ridden to demonstrate the diet skill. Such a bicycle could appear in various flourescent colors with many adornments: bells, horns, balloons, fliers, etc. Furthermore, notwithstanding gibberish instructions over the loudspeaker, this special bicycle must be mastered alone on the diet road (figs. 5, 8).

Strangely, most dieters would get on the crazy seat backwards, grasp the handle bars with their elbows, and endeavor to diet down the road. But of course, most dieters fail (fig. 2). Moreover, no matter how many protean forms this magic bicycle takes, the dieter will fall each time with the standard backwards approach that society promotes. Paramob psychology simply does not foster the requisite **insights** an individual must achieve to attain a mobile diet skill (poem 4). Yet a mentor can teach appropriate *grip* and *balance* techniques to assist in the realization of a genuine diet resolution.

Why are diet resolutions frequently aborted with an orgy of sweets, breads, or fats? The following facts reformulate a wealth of experience with "cheating". . .

- **A** Society won't help.
- **B** Life is tumultuous.
- **C** Civil war is terrible.
- **D** You do what you want!
- **E** There's always an excuse to do what you want to do anyway.
- **F** There is no luck in dieting.
- **G** Seduction is ubiquitous.
- **H** A clear night sky has stars.

At your goal weight, you will grasp that **A-G** have the same inherently neutral emotionality as **H**. The volatile undercurrents of **A-G** for dieters comes from the preeminence of feelings over reason in *fixation of belief*. Taken together, **A-G** constitute most of the excuses diet 'losers' provide. Since 'winning' is not normal, a nascent diet 'champion' would do well to consider these givens at the outset of the diet game (13.210).

The quest for increased beauty starts many dieters. Yet health concerns are often a starting point too. Certainly it is wiser to adhere to a good $12 diet book now than to undergo a $1200 hypertension medical hospitalization, or $12,000 diabetic leg amputation, or $112,000 coronary artery bypass graft complicated by pneumonia and a stroke and expensive rehabilitation in a few decades. Prefer the diet stitch in time to a cardiac suture in the future.

In the beginning you believe you can lose weight. Do you really understand the nature of "fat" itself? Not everybody knows what's fattening or 'poisonous' to dieters. Attaining great knowledge involves pain. Pain-in-reaching is actually good if your vision is on food. Some personal time is required to select the best foods rightly—strictly for your pleasure and health. The right course to diet involves many conflicting dilemmas—civil war. When two neighboring notes (separated by only 1/2 step) compete simultaneously for your attention (to reach or not to reach for the wrong foods) the conflicting notes sound awful (fig. 12); such discord permeates modern music, life.

Waltz through diet days to your own tune as orchestrated by your mentor. His job is to help you survive dietbusters, traverse the void, and write a constitution. You reap the dividends yourself.

Romantic dividends particularly motivate women dieters; it's *glory* for the men. Both sexes want the significant others to appreciate the end result. Given a miserable status quo, to get from low to high self-esteem requires a courageous crusade. The declaration of war against excess fat involves hard-fought redemption, an enhanced state of being, a bright union against a backdrop of eternal darkness...

Poem 1

Eurydice,

    Share my victory over the Maenads. Let my music charm your rise from the peaks of your shadowy cycles of hell.

    Hearken to the luminous cornerstone of our estate. Reserve your spiteful talents for the common cacophony of men, perversion.

    Trust the sacred trace of our courtship, the poetic beginning of our marriage as reflected in our words of love.

Orpheus

CHAPTER 2
RESOLUTION

Suddenly, your simmering caldron of bad feelings about yourself rises up and becomes organized into a psychic tornado that whirls you about on high—your black and white daily images are surrealistically colorized in an appalling frenzy (fig. 8). You land abruptly and resolve to "get back" to a weight you used to be. You want to fret less about trivialities, your plan to pull more within yourself entails a constructive selfishness...

Poem 2

Resolution

Too much I made of future, past
Of things not had, that things don't last
So much I made of not it seems
I lived a life of futile dreams.

I sunder dreams to fleeting larks
And laugh at perfect schemes of game
And focus now on what to do
Just what there is can I pursue
Or cunningly best job for food
Or quietly take in the new
Or privately express my heart
To now myself I do impart.

Consistently better management of *now* over a year is the essence of a typical New Year's resolution. Fake resolutions based only on social cues lack the vital spark that can eventually evolve into starry majesty. The brilliant point of losing weight for yourself is certainly *more pleasure* (plus improved health). You resolve to break out before you break down. Ironically, things usually get worse as soon as you begin to change the heavy status quo for the better (13.203). The psychic pains of processed sugar withdrawl, for example, can cause irritability, headache, shaking, and a sense of malaise. Starting a diet shocks your metabolism—don't do it too much.

Requisites for diet success include: 1) 15 minutes of personal time every day, 2) honest willingness to face reality, 3) guilt feelings about fattening foods, 4) not 'burned out'. Don't deceive yourself by beginning a diet just because you think you ought to do to do something (to assuage your consciousness).

If you merely "wish" to be thinner, then don't diet. Unlike a lottery, there's no luck in dieting (chpt. 1; 13.307). Unlike working for money, power, or glory, acquiring the true diet skill is one of the few great things you can certainly do.

Five typical master graph (mG) outcomes have been plotted on figure 2 for illustration purposes; this figure shows the results when 100 randomly selected people across the nation seek to lose 50 lbs. each. About 55 people will diet on and off for a week or so interspersed by long periods of non dieting (A type). Fifteen slightly fanatical diet aficionados will spasmodically follow each commercial diet fad that comes down the pike (B type).

Fifteen earnest adults will embark on a single diet plan, get discouraged after the second attempt at penetrating their secondary fat zone, and not try again for many years, if ever (C type; tbl. 1). Ten 'rabbit' adults start out losing very fast and then paradoxically 'choke' when pitted against their primal 'dietbuster' (δ type; fig. 9; 13.210).

Only 5 people will lose their primal excess fat, equilibrate at their goal weight, and demonstrate their diet skill has become a submotif of living for them. This high failure rate stems from

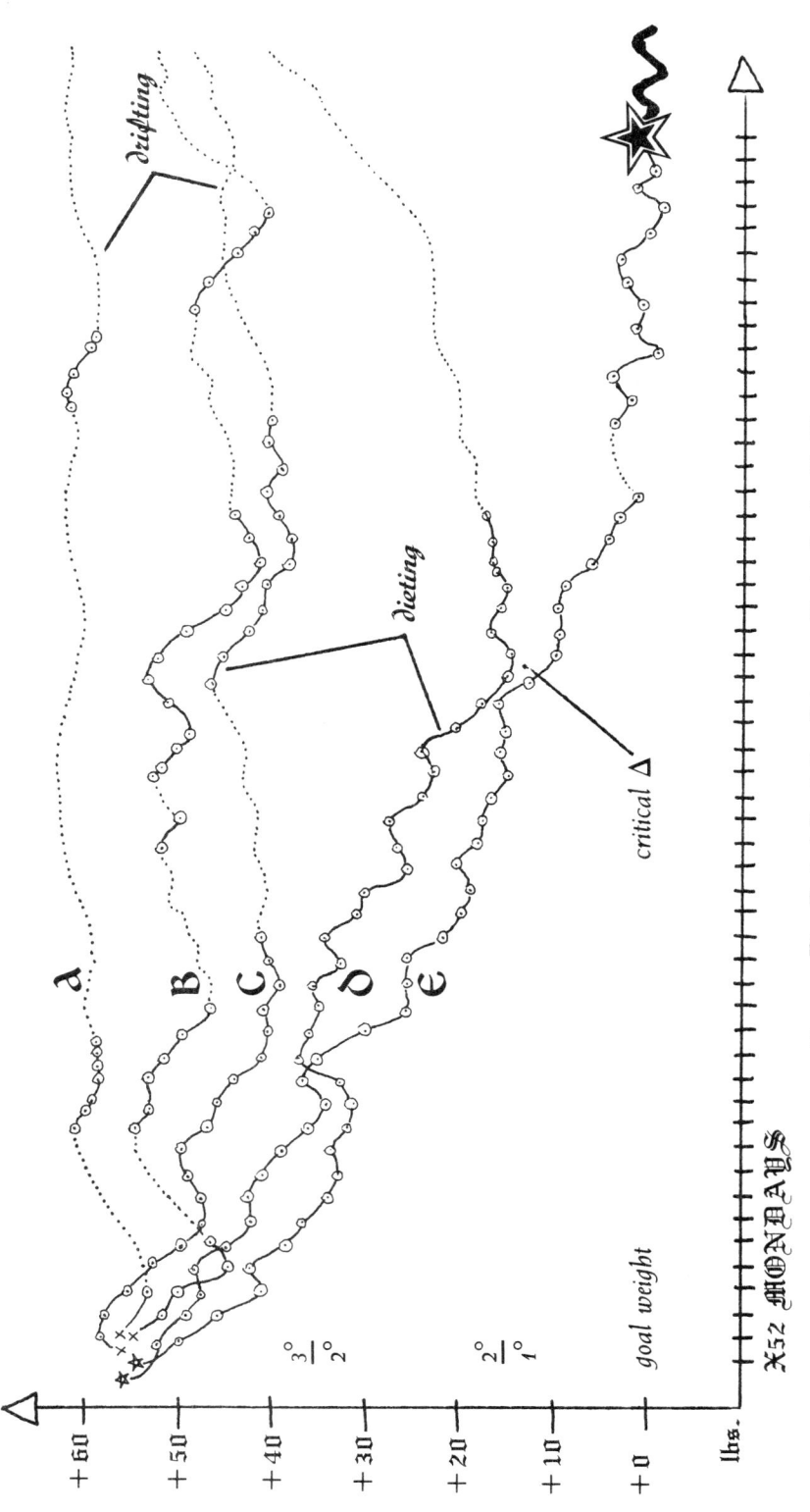

Figure 2. Five Typical Resolution Outcomes, Master Graphs (A–E)

the nature of diet resistances and a general paucity of authentic mentors (chpts. 12, 13).

Compared with this representative national sketch, the star dieter fairs much better. Instead of 5%, approximately 20% succeed outright. This four times greater chance of becoming an ϵ stems from the rigorously personalized format.

Note how curves drift up in figure 2 generally. Overall, dreaded aging constitutes the invisible, relentless arch enemy of dieters. The physiologic decline of aging tends to push your weight up (accelerated by social forces) unless you have an adaptable skill that cancels out each new, silent drop in metabolic rate. The dieter must be as persistent as aging is relentless (seduction ubiquitous).

Figure 3 shows how your invisible baseline (energy used per average square inch of body) declines over a lifetime. Internal and external factors can trigger an inconspicuous, precipitous drop such that eating the same (or even somewhat less through so-half dieting) will net a queer weight gain (beginning of fig. 2C). Obesity is a harbinger of death, the machine winding down, and should be railed against.

Stimulants prop up the machine for awhile (fig. 3). If you stop smoking you may gain a great deal of weight without good diet skills. So if a patient wants to diet and stop smoking, it's best to do the former first. Besides, each form of substance abuse is managed differently.

Surprisingly, will power does not determine outcome. Will power does not exist as commonly believed; rather, virtually all dieters hurl themselves along their diet road once they can envision it through insight (fig. 8; chpts. 1, 6; poem 6).

Nor does the 'spark' for the resolution determine outcome so much as the *mechanism of follow-up*. Familial revulsion or fear may be intense, but it tends to also be fleeting (13.204). It's best to 'piggyback' health onto vanity concerns because social interest in beauty far outlasts that in quality of living; hence there will be more reinforcement for diet work in the sense of enhanced appearances than for philosophical reasons.

Selected aspects of personality actually dominate outcomes. Teachers do best as a group because they often possess the

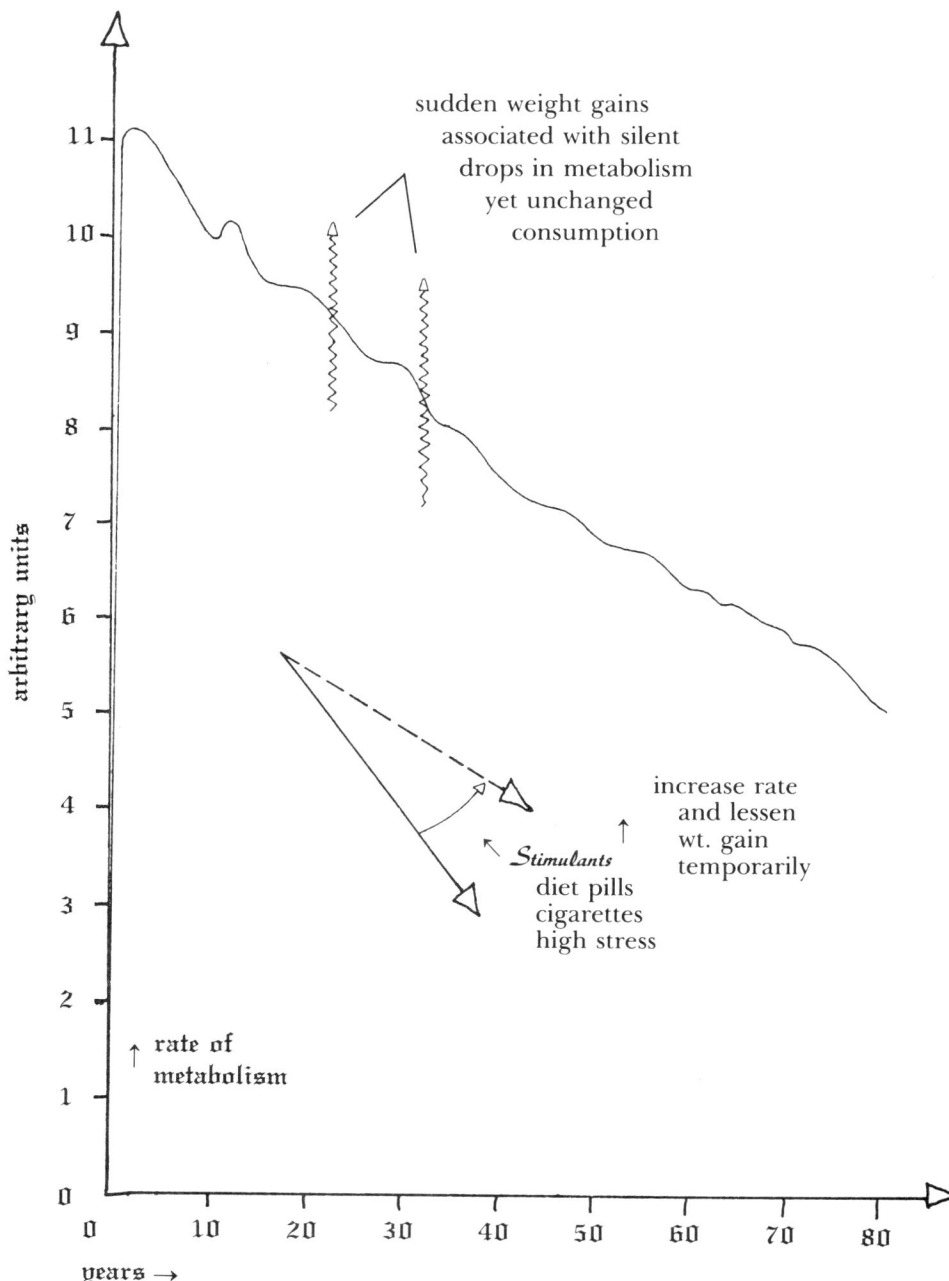

Figure 3. Dynamic View of Aging

intellectual playfulness so very vital to star dieting (poem 17). Anyone that relates well to children has a relative advantage. Other important qualities include **honesty**, motivation, trust, common sense, patience, perseverance and compliance. Somewhat useful qualities include intelligence, irritability, religiousness, independence, or sensitivity.

Chronological age is less important than personality. A lively 56 year old grandmother can possess vastly more youthful thinking (thereby outperform) a dull-witted 19 year old young woman, even though physiologically it's much easier for the younger person. Resolution outcome is directly related to **attitude**.

Learning to diet is like learning to surf the giant waves of aging ("steer" of fig. 1). Stay at the right point, just ahead of the wave, and you'll have a run of conspicuous glory and finish with quiet dignity. Fall into the wrong point, just behind or oblique to the great wave, and you'll lose your grip on the board and be thrown down and about mercilessly in a whirl of negative force (fig. 8).

CHAPTER 3
FAT

"But I don't eat that much!" you say to me. And you were quite possibly dealt a fat genetic card—cursed!? It will require the best of your personality to surmount obesity once manifested as you get older. Of course, "It's not fair" (13.307). Indignation, however does not change how the ancient hands of genetic fate can touch your life, nor how you must eventually pay for your excess pleasures.

Paradoxically, you could view this challenge of obesity as a *blessing* because it affords you a clear-cut way to pitch your *self-esteem* at a much higher level; it's quite rare when you can definitely set your sights higher in life and require no luck at all to succeed. Usually, the heroes of history, besides their talents and perseverance, also needed a hefty measure of good luck to succeed; there's no control over allotments of opportunity, but chance does favor the person ready to make the most out of whatever comes.

So you can cast guilt about being fat out of your heavy emotion wagon (fig. 13). Achilles had a vulnerable heel. Superman fared poorly around Kryptonite. Often your real heroes of history labored against considerable physical, social, or personal handicaps. Napoleon was too short. Franklin Roosevelt had polio. Most people have some sort of mild handicap. Exercises for strength, speed, or the glamor of sexual politics must be done with respect to what you can reasonably do on a day to day basis (chpt. 5). You must start with what you have, from where you are now (poem 4).

Sometimes the handicap of obesity results from disease. Hypothyroidism, familial hypertriglyceridemia or other gene metabolism disorders are occasionally the real culprit (13.307). Check with your doctor if you suspect underlying pathology makes you too fat; such uncommon reasons for obesity are called **endogenous**.

The vast majority of fat people you see on the street are that way because they have not learned the diet skill, which is not to say that they have not dieted nor lack knowledge of dieting; they simply have not learned how to manage their consumption pleasures optimally: **exogenous** obesity. These people store much more fat energy than they use (13.313).

Excess eating is only possible on such a wide scale because humans have learned how to cultivate and distribute food so effectively. You don't need much speed to hunt food in the supermarket, just a fat wallet. In a sense, the food now hunts you through commercial avenues (13.55). There are so many delicious variations to amplify the pleasure effects available through modern vehicles.

Third world countries do not share in our bonanza. WWIII would probably devastate global food availability such that, as in more primitive times, there would be some advantage to possessing high stores of fat in the face of famines (13.308). So in starvation settings, fatness could be viewed as a kind of wealth (as is the case in some African Tribes), a bountiful supply of vital energy.

In Victorian culture the beautiful women had, as a rule, considerably more fat than the so-called beautiful women of today. What distributions of fat (in terms of breasts, waist, hips) are regarded as ideal vary considerably from person to person even within culture today. Certainly, fatness as a sign of disease does not imply beauty at any time. Thus, perceptions of obesity display marked variations through time due to different practical and aesthetic values. So there's no reason, per se, to begin with an overwhelming sense of embarrassment about such a malleable parameter.

Nevertheless, barring apocalypse, you do have beauty concerns that motivate you to better control your level of fatness: **your naked figure** (fig. 1). And once you decide to define for yourself what a reasonably desirable level of fatness you should attain, then guilt about FAT (prominent excess fat far beyond your metabolic needs) does become a useful tool towards cutting it out. You may indeed have had little control over the creation of your 'FAT' state, but once you embark on the diet road, you alone are responsible for the determination of your final state (fig. 8).

Mystically, some of your fetal cells became fat cells; and some more were added in early adolescence. Otherwise, you're dealing with a fixed number of fat cells that collectively get bigger or smaller according to your balance of energy consumed and used over time. Overall, fat cells provide essential sources of long-term energy for daily living: about 20% body fat is ideal.

The relative affinities of breast, hip, or thigh fat cells for the general blood fat that you ingest defines the way your figure is *proportioned*. Like your absolute number of fat cells as an adult, the proportioning of your figure is fairly fixed, so there's very little you can do if, for example, your breasts get smaller faster than your hips when dieting. It's best to do the best you can within the framework of cards you're dealt in life: pass on surgery.

Fat cells themselves are not passive. The bigger they are, the greater their power. Arrowed hormones and nervous messages from FAT will fraternize with primitive brain cells associated with such notions as lust to argue persuasively against continuation of a diet (figs. 6, 10, 12). Fortunately, the hands grip only what the high brain centers command; they can routinely acquiesce to the primitive desires or harken to other high brain ideas for pleasure at will. FAT rules only when the high brain centers have poor inner vision, little insight (poem 6).

Table 1 delineates features at different FAT states. Re-resolutions are particularly necessary at transition points between different zones because the resistances increase substantially as weight drops into the next lower FAT setting. The quantitative approximations of table 1 are a useful guide to determining individual zones even though the exact nature of those resistances have both metabolic and psychological idiosyncracy.

Insight into one's nature, rather than "will power," is a main feature in overcoming FAT; you can not defeat what you can not see (chpt. 6). The general terrain sketched in table 1 does prepare the mind for battle (chpt. 10). Most people begin with

Table 1. Selected Diet Revolution Features at Different Fat Zones

FAT ZONE	EXCESS FAT	STATE	TO ARMS	BY LAND	BY SEA
4	70+ lbs.	gross tomb	despairing	slow walk	placid
3	35-70 lbs.	portly	vicious cycle	fast walk	light chop
2	15-35 lbs.	bothersome	overdoing	jog	choppy
1	1-15 lbs.	annoyance	aging	run	turbulent
0	none ± 3 lbs.	fine *	juggling	routine	calm
−1	−(1-15) lbs.	model	beautifying	climb	whipped
−2	−(15-35) lbs.	cachexia	putrefying	fall	swamp

the simple vision of themselves as just loving "to eat too much;" yet FAT states invariably have latent dietbusters which undermine this peaceful self-view when challenged (fig. 9). Interesting "personality changes" occur when these simple, fun-loving people confront their own subterranean aspects in the fires of craving (poem 1). A mentor should clarify this FAT-nature connection (chpt. 12).

Rather than strive for insight, some people seek surgical solutions to FAT. Typically those that seek dramatically passive solutions reside in "zone 4," the placid one. Wiring the jaws, stapling the stomach, or just cutting FAT out grossly bypass the best way—psychic surgery, sculpting FAT off naturally and artistically (with an eye towards glamor).

Legitimate FAT surgery includes coronary bypass graft, reductive mammoplasty, or fatty tumor excision: necessarily direct assaults on pathological fat. But unnecessarily submitting oneself to a surgeon's knife is an *abomination*. What occurs in the operating rooms won't uplift the spirit generally. Dietbusters are not amenable to physical intimidation (figs. 9,10,11); they tend to be like ghosts in the FAT machine, unperturbed by the conventional wizardry of modern medicine or pseudomedical fad diet schemes (13.60).

Medical management of obesity entails no cutting. Diet pills can be a useful initiating stimulant to get over the initial "hump" if medically supervised (figs. 3, 11, 13). Many drugs indirectly lessen the negative effects of FAT: anti-hypertensives, anti-sugar, and to some extent, anti-anxiety. Often a successful diet obviates the need for any medications in mild disease states. No pills lessen the appetite to the extent that hunger can be avoided entirely (13.320); it's debatable whether such a pill would be desirable, if developed, because of the importance of pain in life (chpt. 5). Diet pills do not eradicate hunger.

Slight hunger while dieting means those fat cells are shrinking—good news! Some pretenders seek diet pills for a "high," physiology does temporarily pick up on watered-down amphetamines, but insincerity has a way of wreaking havoc upon itself in negotiations with the devil (13.303; fig 12). Nearly all medicines become poisons if used improperly (chpt. 4).

A single lowly fat cell stuffs itself with fatty chain energy digested into your blood. You wear the *chains of FAT* forged in life, bite by bite, until you learn how to get one step ahead of aging by adjusting your intake of fattening foods to keep pace with drops in your inherent energy use (fig. 3).

FAT doesn't care about your looks. FAT cares about maintaining or extending its domain. Craving arises when FAT registers anger at dieting (fig. 9). FAT will grow like a cancerous parasite if you let it. Your FAT and your high brain engage in a big war for control of your hands (chpt. 10). Aging (Nazis) allies FAT (Italians) against your wits. You lose if you're not as relentless at breaking the FAT chains because your enemy won't quit (Japanese)...

In the end, even a small chunk of aberrant calcified fat can hit like a sniper's bullet in the chest. Bill, a hard-driving 46 year old insurance executive, closed many a big deal courting clients with rich steaks, wine, and exotic entrees. He regarded himself a connoisseur of good living. His stunning twenty year ascent in the corporation meant his wife and 4 children could live in grand style based on his magnificent persona and resultant income. And he looked the part of a business giant—corpulently adorned in elegant silk suits. His magestic voice resonated a powerful influence at board meetings.

One fateful day he met his foxy mistress at their usual rendezvous. Suddenly a sharp pain stabbed through his chest during sex and he passed out... He awoke in the C.C.U. days after having undergone multiple coronary bypass grafts. His first symptom of fat-hardened heart artery obstruction had been a near fatal heart attack! The stroke he suffered during surgery left him partially paralyzed on the left. His speech was slurred, often unintelligble. He was even incontinent at times: how truly embarrassing!

He'd almost lost the war on the first battle. He'd known he was too fat but since he took executive elevators and didn't exercise; he felt little disability except for getting winded with trivial exertion. Besides, he'd always put off dieting because his manly business concerned him overwhelmingly.

His partners begrudgingly carved up his territory. His mistress disappeared. His wife and children came to visit him with a mixture of pity and terror in their eyes. His net worth plummeted since once routine family living expenses now seemed horrendously high. The omnicient king became a sorrowful liability. His eldest son had to take a job instead of going to college. Eventually he recovered to the point where occasionally he could be taken out to an inexpensive restaurant. He now orders fruit salad, skim milk, and baked fish: too late!

Dietary management of FAT should be done as soon as possible. Desperate dieting late in life may be a harbinger of morbidity or associated with imminent mortality. Learn the sophisticated *hand skill* of dieting in early adulthood (fig. 1). This war with your FAT must be won before the enemy gets too strong. The quality of your latter life may well depend on the outcome.

CHAPTER 4
POISON

Avoid dietbuster 'poison' when dieting. Embrace pure pleasure, nonpoisons, once earned. Poison cautiously becomes nonpoison at your goal weight. All the fattening foods which constitute sin against yourself should be virtually banished until such time that you are constituted to enjoy them without manifestly deleterious effect (fig. 4; 'countersentence'). The practicalities of sin management are not a forte of the church, yet *guilt* sometimes spurs will power admirably...

Poem 3

Invitation

This Christian "courage," reverence bond
Archaic, pallid embers burn.
Do you not query lusting force
Dream songs of love, pure passion's wand
Dark secrets cast without remorse?
Tis precious thrill the best do yearn
From sacred fruits the fearless learn!

Do you harken to devil or saint (fig. 12)? Do you eschew casual chocolate as well as "casual sex"? Seek the higher states of being. Courageous decisions at the main forks in life will make the difference between "571" blessed joys and "10,000 +" damnable obsessions regarding the same pleasure item (fig. 5). A "forked tongue" approach to life may work in social matters, but dishonesty leads to defeat invariably—FAT will not

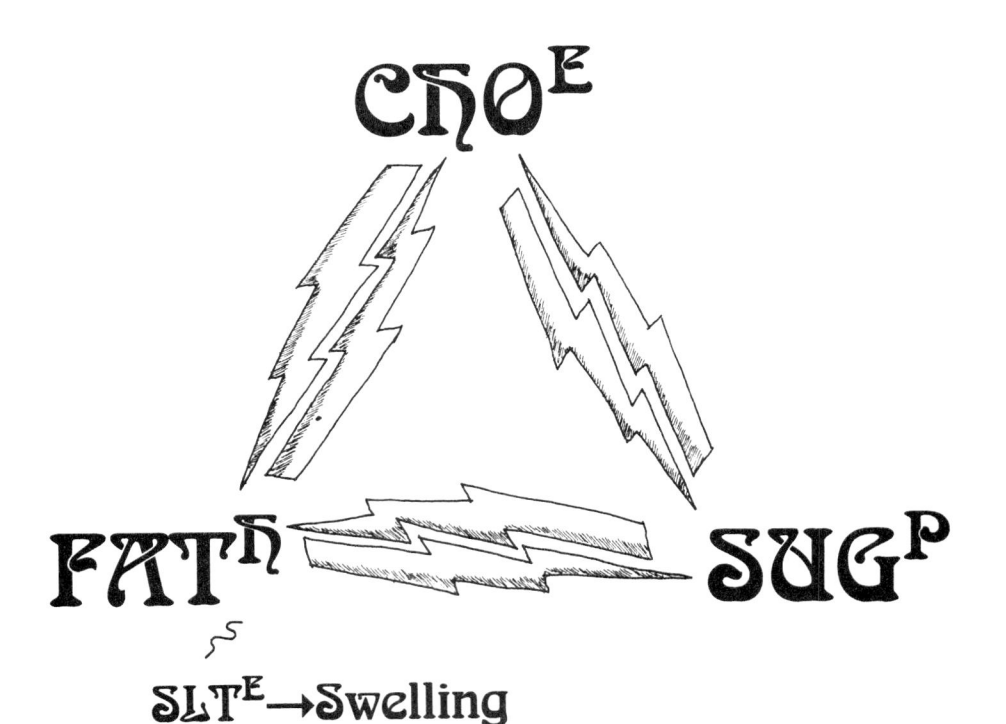

SUG	*FAT*	*CHO*	*SLT*
candies	red meats	breads	chips
pops (regular)	chocolates	potatoes	pickles
ice creams	margarine	cereals	seasonings
"sweets"	"fast foods"	rice	pops (diet)

CHO^E

FAT^h SUG^p

$SLT^E \rightarrow$ Swelling

Figure 4 Lightning Interconversions of Fattening Foods in the Body and the Association of Excess Salt with Water Retention

allow you to "slip around" its self-serving interest and intimate knowledge of what you've actually done (chpt. 3; 13.300).

See the moral analogy between a sweet morsel on the sly and "slipping around" with your spouse's best friend. Illegitimate pleasure eventually manifests as a swollen body, shattered marriage, carnal knowledge: **pagan pleasure** in darkness becomes Christian pain in light.

Setting colors interpretation. Imagine you want a glass of your favorite colored sugar water (red pop), yet you're supposed to be dieting. You know a bottle of red pop would punch a hole in your diet (fig. 11). Nevertheless, it's summer, you're hot, tired, and just "dying" for that marvelous thrill; so you reach for the bottle...

Just before you drink it's whispered in your ear—"Enjoy, for your pop is actually a special wine of godly quality (fig. 12). Never before have you experienced the hundred-fold ecstasies you are about to feel (fig. 6). Though laced with true poison to discourage mortals, you will not taste it in your ravishment. Incidently, you will die convulsively within the hour."

Here a mere **idea** would kill desire. Dieting itself breaks down into a simple series of ideas, strung together to break the shackles of fattening obsession (chpt. 3). The philosophic idea of personal rights, liberty swept across Europe and transplanted in the colonies to incite a revolution. A Declaration of Independence from tyranny can involve breaking with centuries of feudal tradition or years of poisonous values (tbl. 1; 13.203; 13.60). Of course, some compromise will be necessary to win a revolution—you don't need to win every battle to win the war ('C2'). Strategically start with "guerrilla" approach—cut down on fattening poisons as much as you can wherever you can. You do need a little fat, starch, salt, and sugar everyday for nutrition purposes anyway. Keep your resolve on that final state, constituted under God.

False gods have a way of whipping up orgies of frenzied addictions without consideration for ultimate well-being (13.14). Remember, amoral businesses generate siren illusions to lure you to their fattening products. Don't invest in false

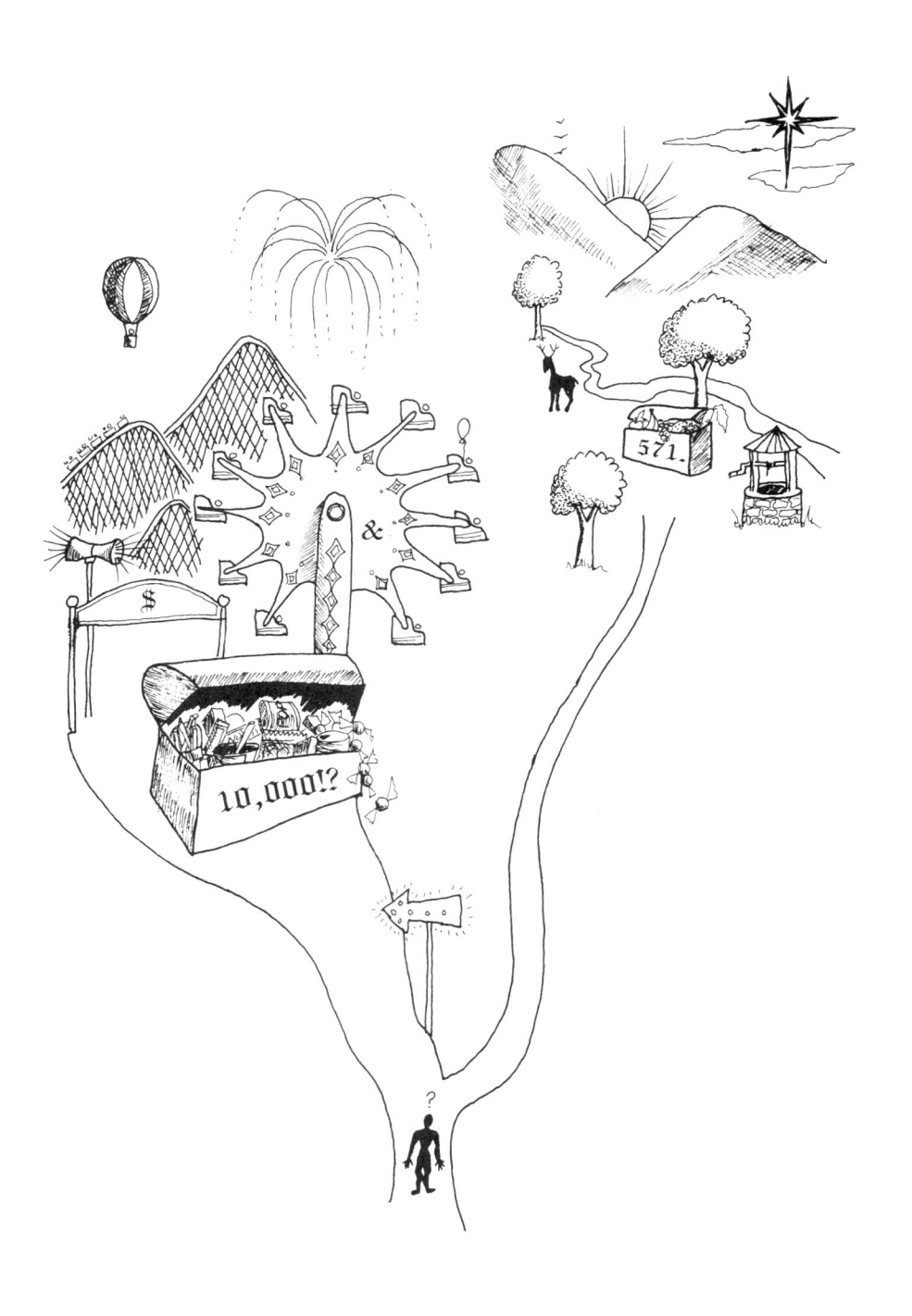

Figure 5. Fork

gold. The many forms of false gold can create the deception of dieting by avoiding only some fattening foods (figs. 4, 10).

Don't deliberately sin against the revolutionary state you have in mind for your weight. Be clever, but not too clever about poisons (13.300). Poison waxes and wanes. Poison to one animal can be food to another. Medicine at one dose can be lethal at another. Sin outside marriage can be just fun within its sanctions. There are many forks in life and since diet always has health ramifications, it's important to generally take the right path. Be respectful of other states, but pursue *your* best interests ultimately.

CHAPTER 5
EXERCISE & POSITIVE PAIN

Life entails pain. You select from a banquet of pain and pleasure; yet roses and thorns come together (frg. 1). Blanket avoidance of all pain sharply limits your access to great pleasure. "Zone 4" people often display low pain thresholds, unrealistic approaches to life (tbl. 1), no diet nor exercise because of the undesirable feelings (13.202, 13.308, 13.317).

If life is essentially a flight from pain, then a modestly logical proposal would be to escape from all pain through hallucinogenic drugs, suicide, or science (13.300). Besides simple addictions, there exists a much more draconian possibility for the future—pharmacologically induced coma (anesthesia) followed by precise electrode placement at brain pleasure centers such that life would become a continuous series of enraptured ecstasies (13.14, fig. 6, 'serial sin'). Gross body maintenance could be performed as for any trauma victim in coma.

Perhaps the body itself would be unnecessary if the brain could be dissected out and kept alive in a large beaker of preservative fluid plus artificial circulation of blood nutrients. Though this ultimate realization of the 'void wish' might please some, one small problem with this electroded heavenly bliss would arise if someone wants to pull your plug (abort): there wouldn't be much you could do about it!

Consistently embracing a little positive pain through daily exercise will yield enduring satisfaction plus probable minimization of negative pain (anxiety, headaches, low back pain, arthritic pain, etc.). Moreover, *satisfaction* directly follows a moderate exercise session when part of a consistent pattern; i.e. the body *wants* and expects this beneficial self-treatment.

The I-can't-endure-hunger-nor-exercise-pain attitude spills into the next day, and the next (13.315). Occasionally you may just feel like exercising but such random inspirations won't carry you throughout a diet (13.317). Prod yourself by playing inspiring music. When you've worn out your invigorated response to specific sounds then evoke primitive "fight or flight" notions. Recurrent nightmares, current fears, and dreadful possibilities in your life can be purposefully used to get your blood stirring.

The **cathartic** advantage of surmounting life's problems in your imagination while exercising can actually benefit real outcomes because of enhanced general attitude. Make sure you do at least token exercises everyday. If you feel bad, do less, but do *something* and record ('$\mathcal{C}_4$').

E* is exercise for yourself. There are 1,440 minutes in a day and very rarely will you not be able to eke out at least ten minutes of exercise. Exercise at least to the point of a little bit of discomfort, positive pain: quickened pulse, sweat between the breasts, aching in some muscles. Don't bound into an exercise regimen like an excited puppy. Do mostly exercises that you prefer; there's no reason not to develop an exercise pattern that's uniquely yours (fig. 1). However, unreasonable expectations will quickly lead to despair. If you overdo today you'll probably hurt tomorrow, negative pain. Life goes on inexorably. Habitual E* prepares you to take the inevitable pains of life more in stride ('positive addiction').

E^s is exercise with a social twist, often considered more fun than E*. One or two times a week play a sport, attend an aerobics class, or simply go for a brisk walk with a friend. These excursions can include a healthy sense of camaraderie or appreciation of nature (fig. 5).

E^w is exercise of work, routine chores. E^w is already calculated into your current weight, so don't point to work on the job or at home as a 'license to eat.'

E* involves no gimmicks, no special equipment, and can be done wherever you go (vacations or trips). Persistent isometrics, progressive pushups, stepping up and down on something, lifting anything a bit heavy for awhile, or dancing in the nude can be done in any private setting. E* goes on regularly, like a heartbeat. E^s relies on joint psychology, logistics, and opportunity; so it can be legitimately cancelled. E* should be a sacrosanct, private ritual (chpt. 11). Yoga is an example of exercise with a spiritual flavor. Develop your own philosophy of exercise. Let your good sense guide a slowly progressive development of E*.

Similarly, stretch your tolerance for hunger. H^c is hunger of craving, a positive pain. H^s is hunger of starvation, a negative pain. Amazingly, if you consistently have 2/4-3/4 the calories in a day you used to eat to maintain FAT then eventually that fraction will appear as 4/4 of what you *want* with H^s at no point. 'Less is more' particularly if the quality of food is higher (13.311).

H^c costs nothing. But a piece of cake typically can be paid for by running a brisk mile: most people repeatedly have the cake and skip the run. Bountifully unused energy gets stored as FAT (chpt. 3). Jog a mile with that cake in mind and you may well think twice about what an innocent piece of cake can mean (fig. 10).

If too much vital energy is devoted to work, family, or social service, then burning off FAT means austere living, dieting with positive selfishness, a prescription for temporary *stoicism* (13.301; 13.60). An important fraction of your total attention must be self-devoted each day.

Ironically, eliminating the dead weight of FAT, though dieting will make you transiently more tired (especially at the outset), will improve your total daily energy in the end. Even a world champion boxer will get mauled if he appears 50 lbs. overweight for a title fight. The *combative* stresses of common daily living lessen with possession of more effective energy (13.201). Your family and work profit indirectly when you master positive pain (chpt. 16).

Exercise involves particular ways the hands move through time and space (fig. 1). As you get older you must wisely coordinate exercise and eating to get a *good grip* on life notwithstanding aging (figs. 2,3). Exercise naturally.

CHAPTER 6
GOOD VISION

First, you must see what is (poem 6). Self-denial of obesity manifests itself as not looking at the scales, not being seen in bathing suits nor revealing outfits, placing those fine clothes that no longer fit out of sight in the dark corners of the closet. Ambiguous clothes that superficially hide your FAT become your routine choice. You strongly prefer that no one sees, especially yourself, how fat and dumpy you've become.

Second, look for **essentials**. High quality food is listed on table two. Most dieters know basic distinctions between the foods listed. Yet adulterated concoctions present in supermarkets require careful label reading to sort out the relative content in fundamental terms. Orient towards the constellation that best suits your long-term desires. Reach for the products that offer you the best value for your life. Shop carefully.

Third, your own hands grasp the helm of your diet ship. You may well be a "team player" kind of person, but diet activity is essentially *solo* (fig. 11). What seductive poisons you do take home will beckon you relentlessly. Your crew may insist on processed sugar but you can still keep it out of sight as much as possible. Turn your eyes from ubiquitous seductions and steer towards your own star, presumably somewhere near the "good" constellation (fig 2; tbl. 2).

Of course, currents of culture, jungle passion, and extraordinary circumstances may prolong your sojourn, yet the basic direction of your destiny lies in the palm of your hand (fig. 1.2). Those that let go of the helm cast their fate to commercial winds and natural drift; they thereby abdicate precious opportunity in life (fig. 2).

Adrift at sea? You view water, water everywhere but you don't want to drink because of excess ions—salts or sugar that

WAT^F

VEG^F FRT^F

PRT^L CHO^S

GOOD ↑ {christian cosmology}

fresh water
fresh fruit
some starch
lean protein
fresh vegetable

&

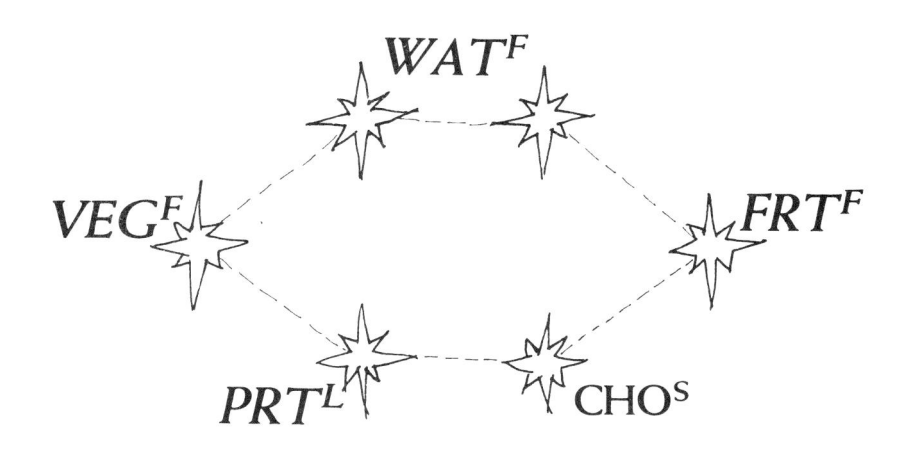

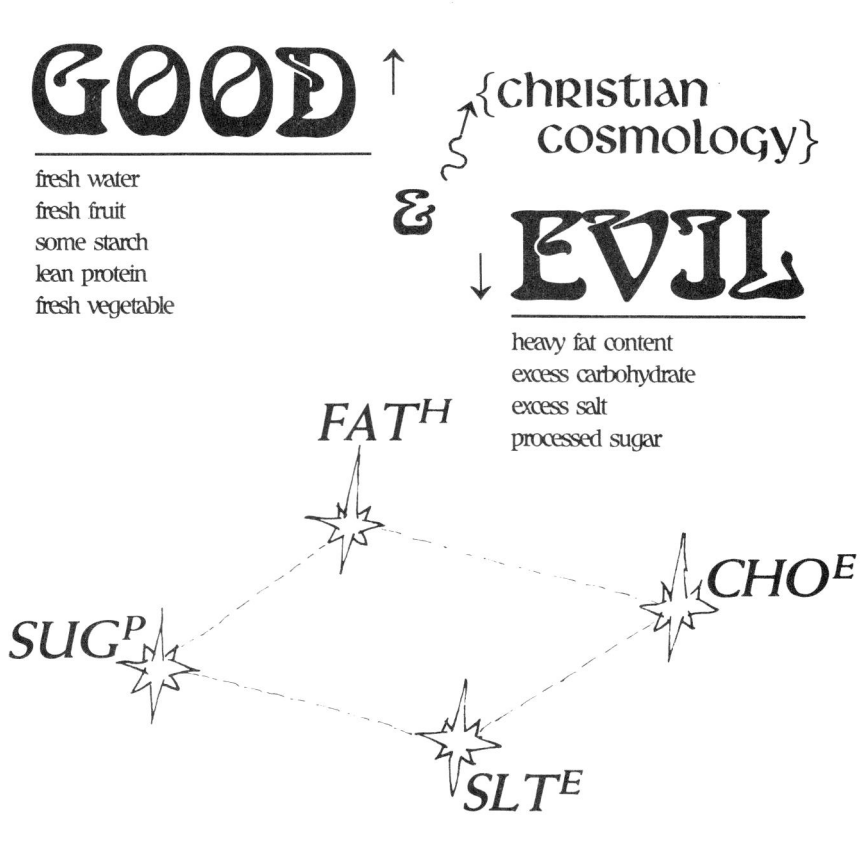

↓ **EVIL**

heavy fat content
excess carbohydrate
excess salt
processed sugar

FAT^H

SUG^P CHO^E

SLT^E

Table 2. Diet Constellations to Steer By

Good Vision

make you just want more (quite profitable for pop businesses, 13.14). It's fresh water that you need. There's plenty of salt naturally scattered through good foods. Fresh vegetables, not loaded with salt, provide important nutrients. Fresh fruit, not punched with sugar, provide vitamins and are a respectable breakfast or snack.

Lean protein, selected dairy products or white meats or low-fat red meats, provide essential amino acids for muscle and metabolism. One nutritious starchy carbohydrate serving, such as some high-fiber cereal or a slice of bread or a few crackers, provide muscle-sparing protection for dieters.

Avert your eyes when you pass through commercial gauntlets (13.55). Break out of the FAT prison that constitutes your wages of sin (chpt. 3; 13.319). FAT imprisonment saps vital energy. Much positive energy is required to see your way out of a black hole amongst the constellation of poisons (poem 1, chpt. 5). The tools of morality can be usefully applied to illuminate the path out of your dark purgatory (poem 1; chpts. 4, 12; 13.200).

The magical road of dieting requires surrealistic colorization of your black and white existence (fig. 8). To get somewhere over the rainbow, one step at a time, mount the scales weekly. Your diet diary becomes the golden currency for the other side (chpt. 11). Keep your sights on your master graph (fig. 2). Take the right fork in the road because you see it's the way you want to go (fig. 5). Use your visionary inner eye to get through the gauntlets of golden glitters. Platonic vision of the *Good* entails a *natural selection* of the best. What Christian would do wrong when they see what's right?

CHAPTER 7
CAVEATS & NEGATIVE PAIN

Learning the diet skill can be extremely important to good health, a **priceless asset**. Maladaptive food behavior has little to do with the average dieter. However, good vision entails extra retinal consideration of the edges of objects since more useful information tends to come from outline than nondistinctive central regions (chpt. 6). We can learn something special from the marginal characters in the diet world (13.323).

Runaway dieting goes far beyond the mild masochistic features of positive pain (chpt. 5). Aberrant psychiatric illnesses do not fall within the scope of a book designed to help normal people overcome small psychological resistances. Serious medical conditions require special medicines, rehabilitation, and diet: *direct* physician care.

Bizarre dieting results from aberrant ideation. Runaway dieting and 'antidieting' are warped mirror images. *Anorexia nervosa* involves extreme aversion to food and typically afflicts amaciated teenage girls with impoverished self-images; these girls fast too much (tbl. 1, "zone -2").

Conversely, the *super-connoisseur* adores food, artfully prepared, and typically traps middle-aged men in their own magnificent zest for high living; such men satiristically mock dieting itself (lords of specious reasoning, 13.300); they question the values of society and cite intellectual arguments via lusty vignettes. Comedians, artists, and salesmen have a high porportion of anti-dieters. Haughty distain for dieting often masks fears (13.200).

The *bulimic* has elements of both anorexics and anti-dieters. The bulimic appreciates food yet vomits it because of self-imaging problems and bad thinking. In *pica* there exists a craving for unnatural foods, e.g. pregnancy or hysteria.

Caveats & Negative Pain

An underlying psychiatric tailspin lands many addicts in hostile lands (fig. 8, 13.14). Diet pills, diuretics, cigarettes, alcohol, and street drugs offer quicksand support to the addictive personality as they sink further into a quagmire. These people harbor psychic monsters that make a dietbuster look friendly (fig. 9). Facing reality is so difficult for substance abusers because of the fantastic screens they put up to confuse intimates, particularly themselves.

Eventually, intractable psychic pain generates defacto negative pain, conspicuous illnesses: depression, migraine, chronic back pain, hypertension, peptic ulcer, diabetes, chronic obstructive pulmonary disease, stroke, cancer, etc. Generally, diet has enormous impact on health, e.g. less cancer of bowel has been linked to high-fiber diets. Your typical doctor specializes in treating specfic sets of tissue pathology from an endless cacophony of diseases. Yet more often than not, the combined effects of personal philosophy and activity have more importance in the etiology and prognosis of disease than medical advice.

Pre-industrial revolution models emphasized the patient telling the doctor what was wrong and needed to be done. Modern medicine precipitated an opposite paradigm—power flowed with burgeoning technology and the rationally "trained" physician became a *demi-god* (13.60).

Now the proper blend is beginning to emerge. Personal values are integrated into the clinical picture, presumably by Family Practice Specialists in particular. Ideally, both the patient and doctor formulate a joint strategy for care. Burgeoning corporate medicine currently complicates this evolution as money and politics pollute philosophical advancement. Revolutions frequently involve changes in ideas associated with money and blood. Men with extraordinary vision tend to lead revolutions.

Contrarily, the addict's vision is bad (chpt. 6); he tends to eventually stagger into negative pain. The regular dieter needs only to take care not to exercise improperly nor to under-eat nutritionally. .

Table 3

Nonideal Approximate Minimum Consumption Each Day to Maintain Health

fresh water	3 cups
fresh fruit	1 cup
starchy carbohydrates	1/2 cup
lean protein	1 cup
fresh vegetables	1 cup

Obviously, active disease states require close, direct medical supervision. Seek out your local physician when negative pain arises in your life. Some people simply cannot pursue their inner destiny alone. Seek appropriate professional guidance when you need help.

Returning to the theme of romance, raising your level of femininity through star dieting may well attract men or spur jealousies. Realization of any *fantasy* may yield a state far worse than the original perception of deprivation and unfulfilled dream. Thus, the most sinister of caveats is represented by the treacherous serpent in the Garden of Success (fig. 10).

Evoking your primal desires from the depths of your being may bring forth far more than just will power for dieting. You can never be entirely sure the forces of unadulterated intent, once manifested, won't change your life irrevocably; yet often this is precisely the underlying purpose of the diet (13.00).

Atomic energy mimics star power; it can be used for peace or war, towards utopia or oblivion, dreams or nightmares ('🌀'). Unleashing the naked potential of your spirit may generate more power than the delicate nature of your current relationships can accommodate (13.205, 13.64). A star can be serenely satisfied or sadly solitary in its glory, as admired from afar. . .

Poem 4

Warning

Ancient purveyor of life's nettled ways
I fathom spring love as you feel it—
Reborn from fatty familial matrimonial maze
(Once tumbled deftly from one aspect to the other)
Suddenly seared slim, so now your pristine passion
   phase.

Emergent beauty, naked resplendency
Impaling duty, enchanting tendency
Stark passion burns in your bones
Empty arms, aching heart, addled mind
The kind that can not find peace alone, but must
Land thy fresh fleeting hope on grounds of lust
Made tranquil by tormenting tease and tyranny:

Tis cursed or blessed that follow me
I know not which but caution thee.

CHAPTER 8
SEX & FOOD

"I love chocolate" makes sense because you're wired for sex and food. **Pleasure** unites these basic drives irrevocably (fig. 6). As a social primate we tend to pursue basic wants within the context of intimate relationships that also give much security. The language of sex and food are intertwined romantically...

Fragment 1

Timeless

Precious love, you beckon me!
You call me forth to champion your survival
   to bleed from your thorns
   to taste your sweet nectar
You submit to my will and thirst for my
   "power."
You fire my spirit, caress my manhood,
   brighten my universe
You capture my heart with your nakedness,
   your virtue
You sign your name to mine with the
   essence of your soul.

The politics of love has undeniable *mutuality* but no true democracy. The state of enduring existence at goal weight means the balanced marriage of inner desire and external control. Proper hand movements demonstrate this balance (fig. 1).

Sex & Food

Women tend to reach for *romance*, whereas men grasp for the *sex*. Phenylethylamine rises after sex or chocolate (fig. 6).

Disturbances in sexual politics cause misery; and in despair, many people turn to food for solace. Alternately, in jubilation many people turn to food for celebration (chpt. 9; '℃$_a$'). It takes time to learn how to juggle the important parameters of life. The life you learn with may well not resemble the life you lead afterwards, hopefully much better given a tincture of wisdom. The quality of living can often be deduced by the caliber of hand skills mastered and the values implied.

Animals seem instinctively preoccupied with pursuit of food yet also devote crucial time to mating. Primitive "romance" focuses on *discriminating courtships*: appearance (e.g. figure, color, clothes, hairstyle, make-up), smell (e.g. perfume), sound (e.g. intonation, discourse), and timing (e.g. opportunity, predispositions, setting).

Overall, food-time far exceeds sex-time for both humans and animals; yet humans devote much time to direct and indirect romance (flirtation). The direct payoff for sex and food is similar: content relaxation (fig. 6). The longterm values of sex and food are children and living respectively. Existence of our species depends on both of these "mixed blessings" (chpt. 10).

Relaxation in sleep dominates nearly a third of living. Sleep time surpasses combined sex-and-food time for most people of advanced countries. Night dreams are too often forgotten (☺). Day images absolutely dominate common free thought in modern society: commercial desires for money, power, or possessions. Thus T.V., movie, or game show images play off these conspicuous interests; and advertisers can subtly link latent sexual interests to cars, toothpaste, or computers. After all, many nouns have gender.

Diet to re-ignite *other* pleasurable interests. Nobody voluntarily gives up pleasure unilaterally. "Will power" does not mean masochism (13.309). Embracing positive pain does not necessarily lessen pleasure, even short term. The trick is to gradually develop nonfood pleasures as you slowly diet. Frantic consumption of "fast food" sickens the soul, addicts the spirit to diet poisons. Learn to appreciate good food the way you would

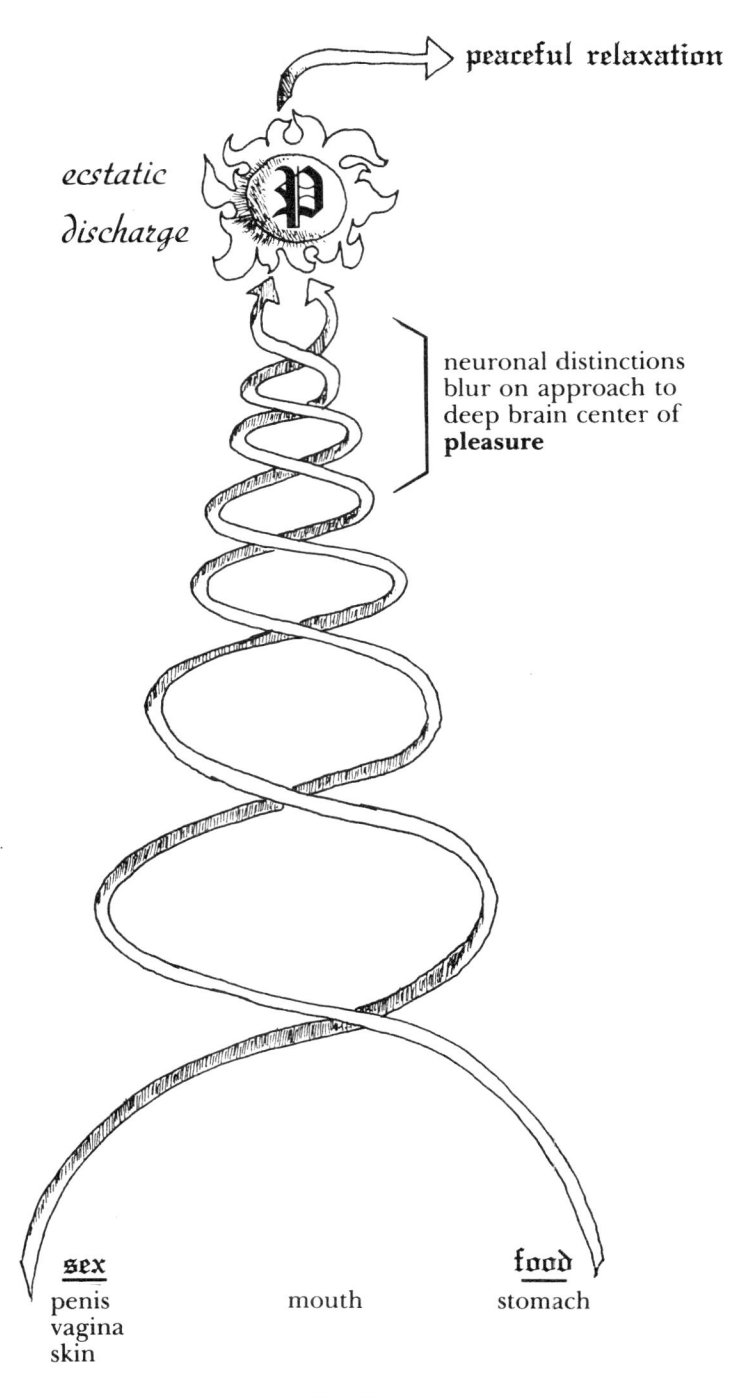

Figure 6. High Wires

if you'd been truly starving. Use the diet flame to rekindle exquisitely personal interests concomitantly.

Explore your interests as well as your body (fig. 1.2). Nonfattening pleasures include art, sport, hiking, craft, literature, music, sex, etc. Take a special interest in children. Many imaginative derivations of these pursuits exist. If you're riding a bike it's doubtful you're also eating a sundae. Having fun while dispensing positive energy is the legitimate concern of all life—not just childhood.

Make sure you have 3 regular, small feedings of good food at your 3 hungriest times every day (fig. 7). Of course, arrange these feedings according to your own schedule, but space them out and don't skip (e.g. 7:15am, 12:30pm, 6:45pm). A mere apple may be considered a minimal feeding, though generally amounts will not be an issue so much as the **nature** of the food you're having (tbl. 3). Avoid eating just because you're hungry. You want to somewhat dissociate hunger and consumption while dieting (chpt. 5). Just limit yourself to regular feedings and possibly a small snack. Note 'deviations' honestly ($\mathbb{C}_2$).

Alternating various lean red and white meats each night helps some "meat-lovers" get their protein without too much monotony. Many diet books provide copious examples of ways to reshuffle the nonfattening food deck through imaginative recipes (chpt. 15). Be careful not to be lulled into the specious reasoning frequently engendered by such books (13.312, 13.313, et. al.).

Fundamentally say "no" to the wrong forks in the diet road until you're positioned to go either way for pleasure without deleterious effect (fig. 5). Pursuit of natural mixes of needed food and special delicacy parallels good discrimination in sex. "Casual sex" implies a low level of discrimination and invites untoward consequences like V.D. or a turmoil of intimates (fig. 8). Since actual sex itself has sharp physiologic limits due to its intensity, only romance can greatly extend the meaning of sex through time: love.

Just as the eyes reveal the soul so do hand actions reveal intrinsic morality. In fanatical Islam the hands are cut off for thievery. Star dieting lends romantic meaning to food deci-

THREE REGULAR, SMALL FEEDINGS FROM THESE GROUPS...

1. **FRT**$^{F(4.)}$ apple, grapefruit, pear, bananas...

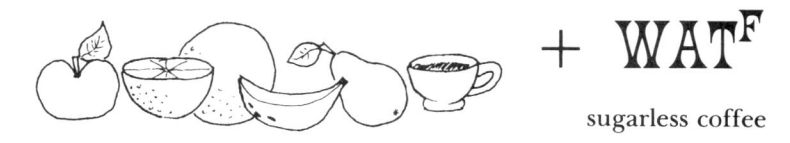

    + WAT^F

    sugarless coffee

2. **SALAD** lettuce, tomatoes, carrots, celery...

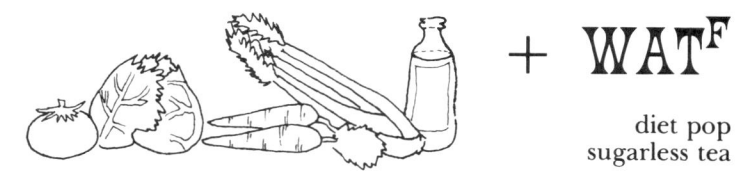

    + WAT^F

    diet pop
    sugarless tea

3. **PRT**^{L}/**CHO**^{S} white meat (red), bread, veg...

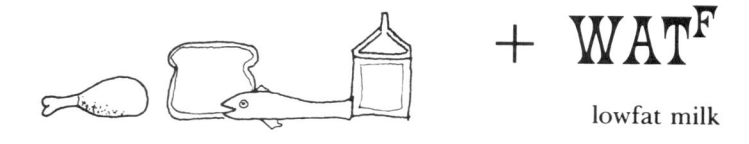

    + WAT^F

    lowfat milk

Figure 7. Sample Ideal Dieting Day

sions. Carnal knowledge of quality sex mirrors direct knowledge of quality in food. Addictions to low caliber pleasures lead to despair (13.14).

The aggressive territoriality of sexual politics interplays with deep-seated **lusts**. A *prescription for happiness* is to bring true want, need, and possession into close practical alignment.

CHAPTER 9
PERSONAL TIME

"Good times" mean fine food, joyous excitement, and often, good sex (chpt. 8). Money earned by slavish months of hard work gets readily spent on happy days. Generally, the way "personal time" is handled clearly reveals the basic values of a person. Star dieting involves learning how to youthfully play with personal time with an eye towards adult *intention*.

Earlier this century physicists proved time bends. You can do what you want with personal time in many senses. Contour your body to its best possible dimensions, particularly during unstructured time (13.51). The success of a diet depends on using your hands to bend, twist, or tailor consumption to improve your figure "forever," like true love—enduring (figs. 1, 2; frag. 1; poem 14).

Only 15 minutes per day of conventional time are required to succeed at dieting. There's nothing necessarily hectic about the clock hands you were taught as a child. Only 1% of your 1440 minutes each day is needed to get to your goal weight. Thus your actual time investment needn't alter your social obligations.

Burst the wrist chain of slaving after time, like the frenzied "white rabbit": always late, always too busy, no time to exercise, eat right, nor live greatly (13.301). The false gold wrist watch pays tribute to Cronos, God of Time and your primitive universe. Strip off the chains of FAT you forged in life, bite by bite, day by day (chpt. 3).

Expand personal time universally! Two conventional months equals a diet week (13.313). One conventional week equals a diet day. Reverse the implosion that occurred with adulthood. Develop the habit of wrestling free for at least some time every day. Align your time not with just our tiny solar system but also with the blasting apart universe of stars. Make room for personal growth and the evolution of your destiny. Regard your mG with the same loving care as a grower of plants. Patience and the long view are paramount (chpt. 10). Climaxes come about more slowly with diet activity, but can be much more enduring than more quickly derived pleasures (figs. 6, 13). The "irrational" universe has plenty of space, a private star for everyone on earth.

Proceed both backwards and forwards in time. Rekindle childhood willingness to acquire new psychomotor skills (fig. 1). Advance your use of feelings towards the future (C_a). Eventually, carefully woven strands of confidential time can constitute an invisible screen against conventional interference (13.50).

"Twilight times" such as weekends or vacations are just a fraction of the total gamut of real opportunity. Between the chores of living there exist cracks of time when virtually any thought is possible. Being immersed in the glaze of T.V., hour after hour, promotes erosion of dynamic character. Current modern media benefits humanity by reducing intercultural distances with entertainment or information, but harms by tending towards abject banality or sophisticated gossip. Evolving character needs quality time based on the true potentiality of the individual. There's generally far more potential for personal joy by actively **doing** what you like than by passively absorbing fantasy rays from the T.V. A star puts out its own rays.

Expanding thighs, bulging abdomen, and increasing clothes sizes imply fat cell growth as a function of aging, increased passivity, and a declining personal universe (fig 3). Railing against the horror of FAT is the diet war (chpts. 3, 10).

Timing is the crucial element of attack in a close civil war, either side can win; and momentum proves a pivotal aspect of conventional mock war outcomes (e.g. basketball, football, baseball). The modern gladiators that consistently create winning momentum for their teams by making "big plays" are heroes, "stars"; such champions typically set up these big climaxes by long and hard practice—constructive use of their personal time beyond the call of practical duty.

E* self-teaches the value of one minute, just as years of tournament golf self-teaches the value of one stroke. The hacker will take "easy shots" for granted that the champion will not (13.210). An additional minute of exercise, boldly going beyond easy self-limits, elevates your morale and vastly improves efficiency for the rest of the day (chpt. 16). Those few extra leg lifts, push-ups, or yards jogged can illuminate personal being; it's precisely at these key moments when you "don't feel like it" that the greatest gains are possible (13.317). Life usually turns on very brief moments of critical difference (fig. 2).

There's nothing wrong with quick bursts of cheap pleasure. Figure 5 implies that "571" of such pleasures within a natural time frame is ideal. Hence the distribution of casual pleasures sparingly over time affords the best blend of good and evil (tbl. 2). Star dieting is civil war between relative good and evil, designed to accomplish a subtle, significant shift away from passive pleasure and towards more active pleasure. The pressures of modern living can seem to slowly strangulate *fun*, personal time. You must fight to keep the most cherished dreams of childhood alive, evolving in space and time.

Sharpen your sword of personal values and sculpt FAT away, banish. War is art too. The point of enduring the inner strife of dieting is attaining that lasting sense of tranquility and beauty that typifies our image of a star.

CHAPTER 10
CIVIL WAR

The *turtle* is the animal of inspiration in your civil war of dieting (fig. 13). Conflict rages between one hand that would reach on impulse for any convenient pleasure and the other hand that would carefully discriminate among pleasures with respect to your goal for your naked body (figs. 1, 12). Only slow, patient "evolution" will yield the best organism possible. Personal resistances vary enormously, progress occurs in a unique emotional milieu.

Extraordinary adaptions in nature illustrate the dramatic results of small changes over a long time in developing the fantastic characteristics of some individual species. Certain Galapagos lizards do not seek insect food in the deserts; they have learned instead to dive in the ocean, swim along underwater and eat algae off the rocks.

Some acacia plants actually house and feed ants which, in return, devour other insects that would eat its leaves. Venus fly trap plants, rather than rely on defensive allies or poisons, offensively "eat" insects by closing shut rapidly with hair-trigger fury. The blue-footed fishing birds of the Galapagos Islands dive gracefully from the sky into the water and catch fish; whereupon specialized frigate birds often attack and pirate prey away from the blue-footed fishing birds.

Magnificent geological formations—canyons, waterfalls, mountains—as well as great human accomplishments—The Great Wall of China, The Pyramids of Egypt, the trips to the moon—all come about because of much slow change or persistent force towards some ultimate effect.

The hare, in contrast, is fast, impetuous, and arrogantly inattentive at times: a loser (fig. 2ծ). The tortoise is patient, steady, and genuinely humble: a winner (fig. 13).

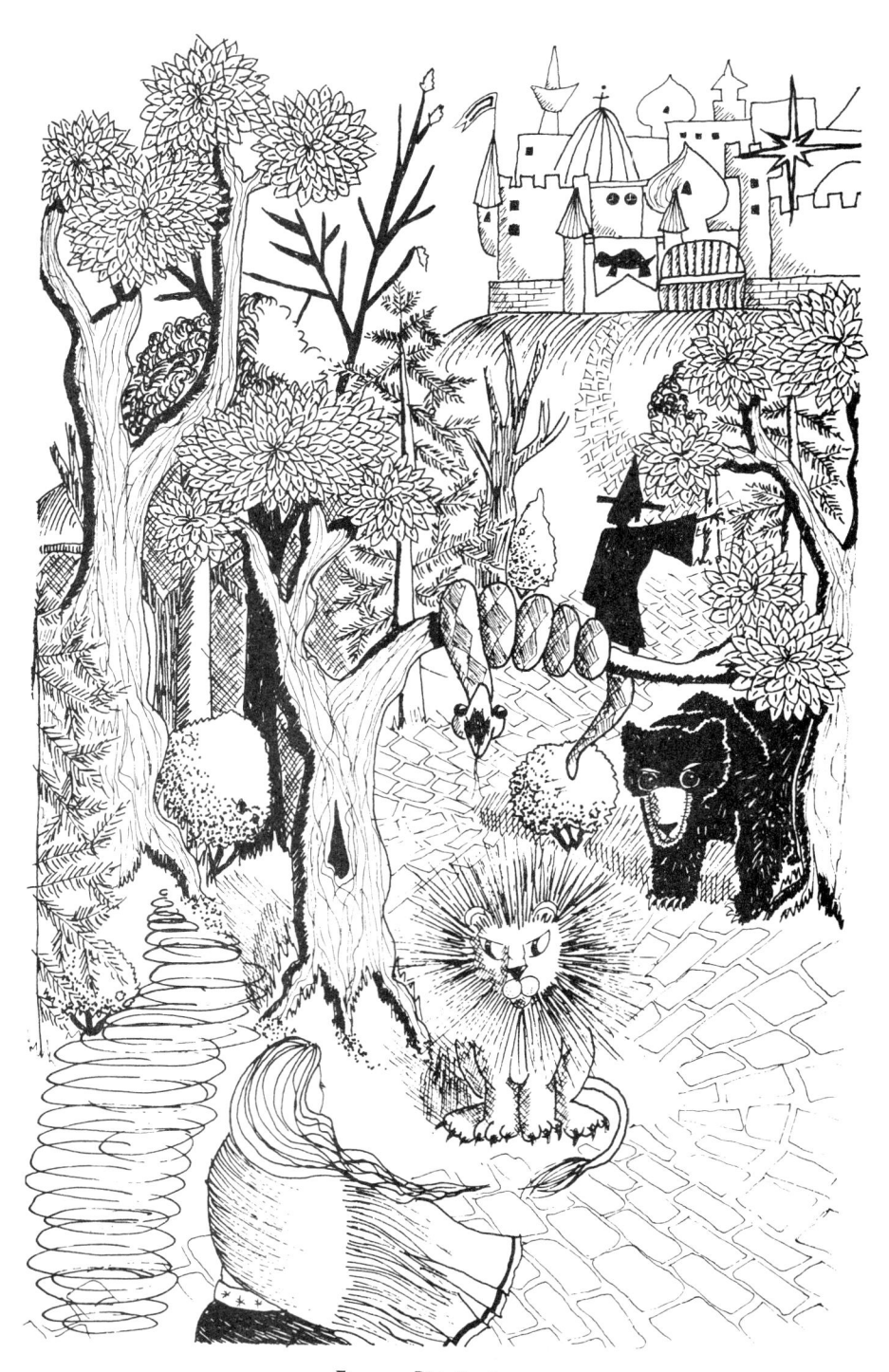

Figure 8. Diet Road

Civil War

So if a *tumultuous* tornado of life has landed you in an unhappy place and you want to go home (to what was before yet would be better upon return) follow the diet road to your desired state of weight patiently (chpt. 9; fig. 8). Expect problems and delays in your great journey. Look for a mentor, not a wizard's wand that would suddenly put you back to your previous weight. Without key insights (e.g. "there's no place like home," chpt. 16) your weight would just insidiously rise again. Stress, pregnancy, and aging behoove one to develop a major skill—the adaptation of diet. You don't have to eat algae, nor insects, but baked fish is not such a bad idea.

Expect to encounter frightening creatures along the surrealistic road of dieting; some little ones you can shoo away, some will annoy but not impede, some may turn into courageous allies or instigate useful notions (e.g. "fight or flight" prompts to exercise, chpt. 5). At least one creature will have to be killed outright. Usually, a wicked Queen of Hearts or Witch of the West appears during primal excess weight loss; yet these forms of the **devil** may present themselves in an infinite variety of draconic images: jealousy, impatience, anxiety, boredom, mirage, etc. (tbl 1). Beware of the dietbusters and their protean forms (figs. 9, 10).

The climactic battle with the witch must be won or the war is lost (fig. 2☽). Of course, quitting can come ingloriously at any point for a "summer patriot" (13.303)...

The soldier had miserable rags for shoes in subzero winter, a rusty old musket without ammunition, scant food, a crowded makeshift shelter through which the winter winds howled; and he saw no prospect for any victory to end this cursed Revolutionary War. He thought, "Why not just slip out of camp when the sentry falls asleep? I could be enjoying hot biscuits and gravy back home with my family within the week..." How bizarre the summer fanfare of a diet resolution seems when compared with the wintery waves of without: wanting.

Stone cold aging blows invisibly (figs. 2, 3, 8), a *relentless* enemy that you can engage only in the twilight zone between your light and dark sides (13.200). *Vexation* often means progress yet promotes desertion. Dreams are useful arms in a war

Figure 9. Composite Dietbuster

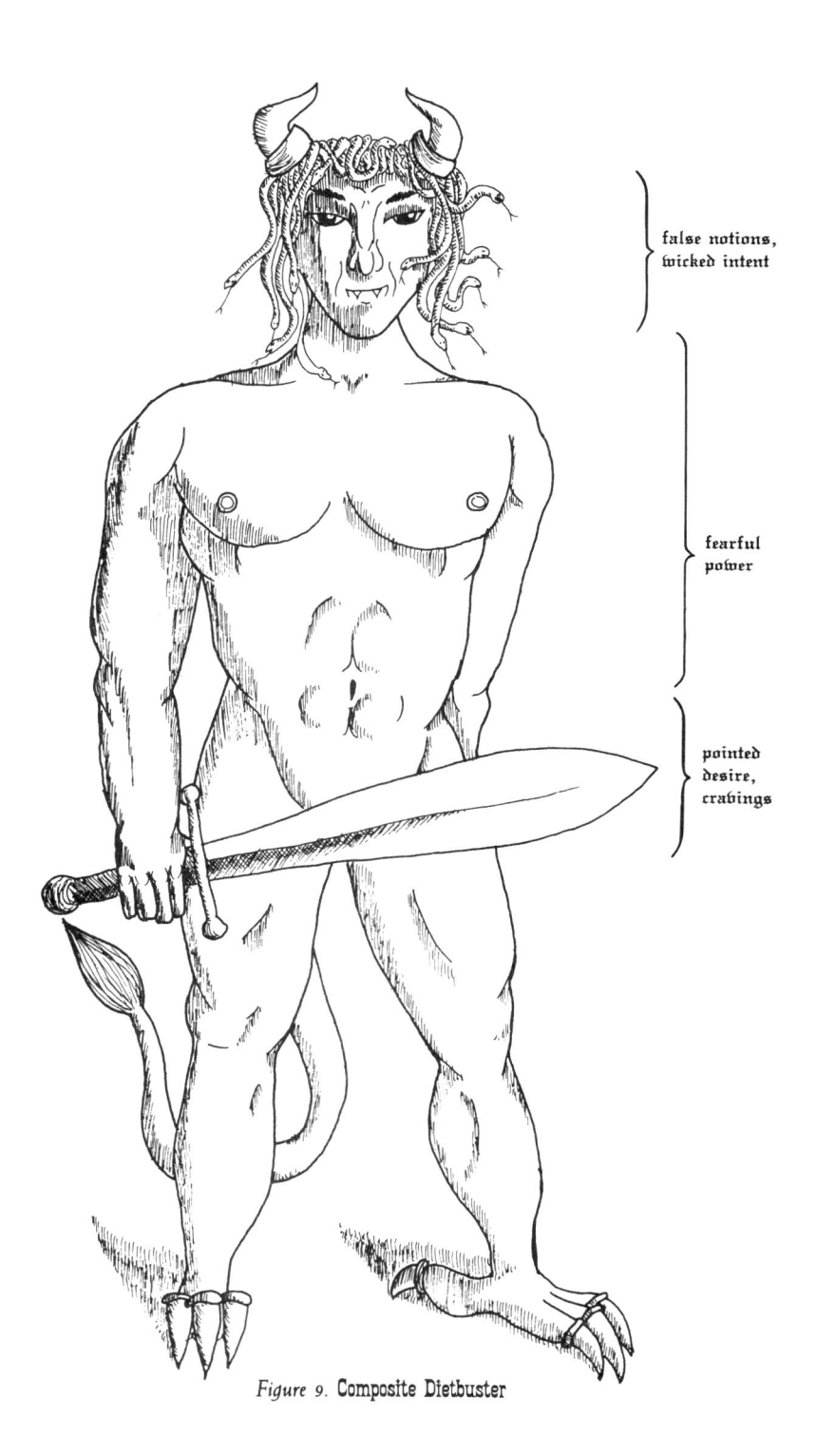

- false notions, wicked intent
- fearful power
- pointed desire, cravings

between inner spirits (ⓓ). Hope and will power may well enter through dream windows or from the bottom of Pandora's Box.

Every battle needn't be won to win your civil war (ⓒ$_2$). Grind out each little victory you can (ⓒ$_1$). Continue with scathing honesty. Harken to battle hymns (poems 1, 14, 15). Finish courageously (13.210). Spend some time framing your new constitution (chpt. 15). Keep marching to the music of your destiny.

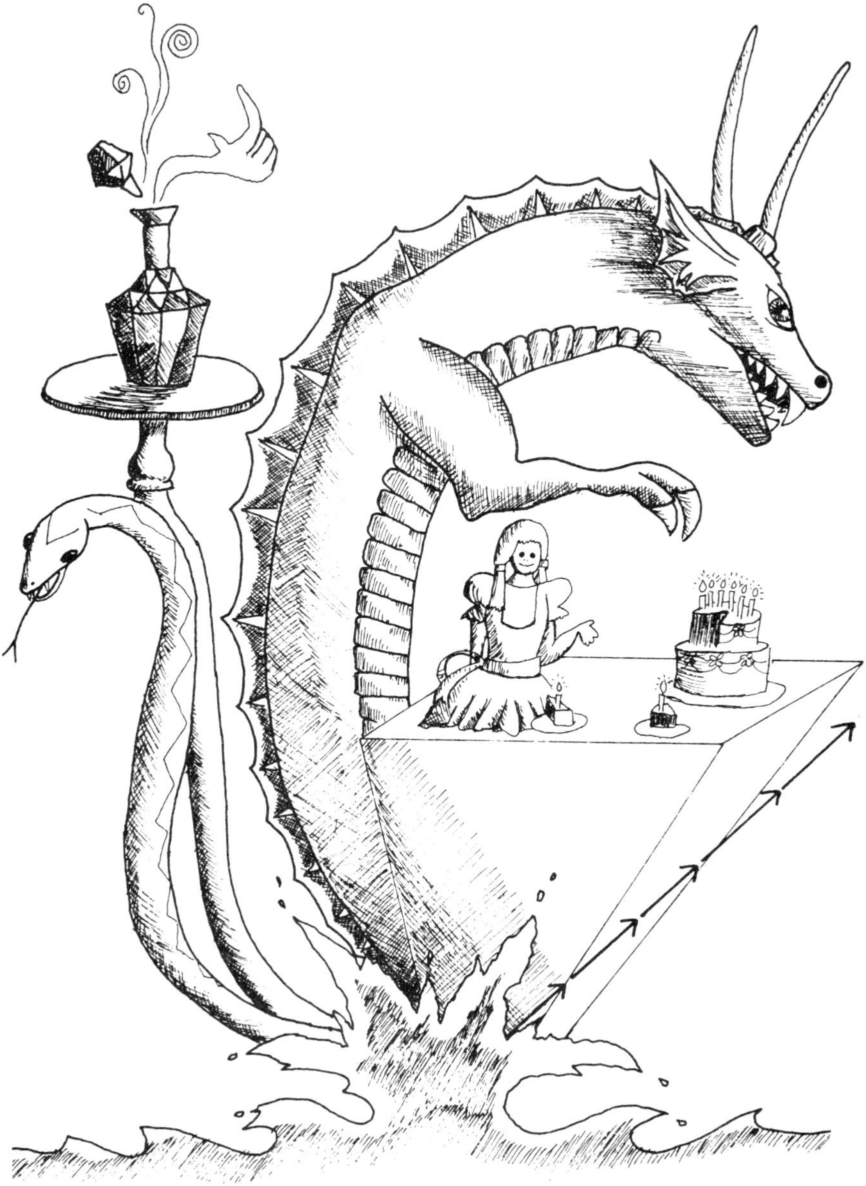

𝔖inister ambush, evocative summer wine, hunger dragon, birthday cake, hormone arrows amongst tumultuous diet waters.

Figure 10. Protean Resistances

CHAPTER 11
DAILY WALTZ

Let the virginal, upbeat beginning of every diet day be to caress your naked body before a mirror and write the day and the date in your 'diet diary' (☉☉; frg. 2). A sculptor uses hands directly to create nudes out of excess clay. You work intimately with your FAT. Both the mind and the *hands must focus on the artistic objective*. This arising ritual tends to mitigate specious reasoning for the rest of the day (13.300).

Table 4

Waltz Step Equations

$1 = \text{'PPP'} = \text{'P'} + \text{'B'} + \text{'D'}$

$2 = \text{'DP'} = \text{'EF'}$

$3 = \text{'PP'} = \text{'C}_1\text{'} + \text{'C}_2\text{'} + \text{'C}_3\text{'} + \text{'C}_4\text{'} + \text{'C}_5\text{'}$

The purpose of private twilight dances between the light and dark phases of your life is the evocation of the primordial currents of your being (13.309). Morning ritual (PPP) consists of activation of the body with respect to naked desires or dreams. Daily ritual (☉P) consists of immediate execution of the facts of consumption (EF). Nightly ritual consists of a systematic series of comments designed to conjure a crucial critique (C).

Incisive new rituals are required to replace entrenched fattening ones. Drive a magical wedge between the sanctity of your sleep and doing whatever for whomever else, such as grooming for society or going to the kitchen for food or drink (e.g. coffee stimulant). When your eyes open act (P) first for yourself: look at your naked body (B) while reaching back for your dreams (☉; fragment 2; poem 10); briefly sketch any dream fragments you recall in your diet diary (fig. 13). Add any feelings or perceptions about your changing naked form as well as any *re-resolutions* about what you intend to do about that form. Activate (✍) your diet diary by writing the "day" and the "date" to symbolize culmination of the morning ritual. Days of the week have different challenge levels, weekends are nearly as difficult as holidays (13.51).

Children act more with respect to their imaginations than adults; but "magical thinking" carries into adult life, especially as superstition. Each morning you should at least glance at your mG and consider how you'll look at that projected star point and what 'seductions' will likely arise that day. Dieting should be both exciting and productive in the best sense of childishness. In order to get one step ahead of aging (instead of one step behind, i.e. FAT) it's vital to be scathingly honest and direct in your diet diary because aging can not be "faded" nor reasoned away (fig. 3).

Some adults are accustomed to shading the truth a bit for the sake of expediency (13.300). Yet constructively honest "child's play" is the creative essence of impudently fashioning a body against the flow of aging, society, or pregnancy. Children display not only more frankness but also tend to pay for their sweets with much more active play, exercise (chpt. 5; 13.316). Dream writing may prompt childlike visualization of dietbusters because formal specious reasoning doesn't exist in dreams (figs. 9, 10).

Write all that you eat or drink, 100% honest, as soon as possible after consumption. Take your diet diary along with your naked body, i.e. everywhere you go. It only takes a few moments to jot down exactly what you've done. You're interested in getting a secure grip on what you actually do (fig. 1.3). Many dieters think rightly and do wrongly. Letting go of the helm and punching holes in your diet with 'deviations' usually sinks your diet ship (fig. 11). Omit nothing, estimate, write details exactly: #'s (especially deviations), cup fractions, oz's, additives (13.315).

Consistently honest recording in your diet diary far outweighs "will power" over the long haul (fig. 13). You may use a tiny Asian import pen to record your thoughts in a conveniently small diet diary. **"Pen and sword in accord"** refers to an ancient Japanese insight, useful for the spirit of your diary writing. The further you progress, the more important the diary component becomes (fig. 13). During 'phase III' all such writing may taper to nothing.

Before sleep, take advantage of your secure grip on your actual deeds of the day by commenting upon them. Victories ($ⓒ_1$) and defeats ($ⓒ_2$) involve your net hand movements relative to the major seductions of the day. Feelings color the main emotional events of the day (fig. 8). Overall, reactions to feelings dominate outcomes (chpt. 2). Exercises recorded as done mean far more than exercises you intended to do or sessions you signed up for but never did. Gauging the final hunger level indexes your relative accomplishment far better than counting calories (13.313).

$ⓒ_1$ is victories. Society will deliver temptation to your fingertips and sometimes virtually insist you indulge. Skirting the consumption part of a spontaneous office party, pausing at the candy section but moving on while shopping, driving by that fast food franchise you used to frequent daily, going for a nice walk at the family reunion picnic at just the time when deserts are being served, taking your children to Wonder Delights ice cream store on a hot summer day and driving out with only diet slush in your belly, watching your family eat your favorite desert (that you made and served) yet having none yourself, or sitting home alone and ignoring the beckoning cry of those chocolate chip cookies in the cupboard—all illustrate saying "no" to diet poisons (chpt. 4). A string of victories usually wins a war (chpt. 10). Good soldiers should be decorated fairly soon after an heroic act (chpt. 12).

Partial victories deserve comment too. Having one piece of pizza instead of three, eating only half of a candy bar instead of all of it, or only tasting a deviation instead of gorging yourself— all illustrate an accomplishment worthy of notation. Try for at least partial victories every day, even when compromised by adverse circumstances.

C_2 is defeats. If the left hand reached for a forbidden treat and the right hand failed to slap the left away, then a 'deviation' occurred (fig. 12). Write a formal excuse for each deviation and include setting, feeling, and judgement along with the explanation "I had *xyz* deviation today because. . ." Setting involves who, what, where, when, why, or how. Your feeling at the time of ingestion is relevant. Did you feel this deviation was justified? It's quite a drag to relate to fattening food this way, just the act of writing any kind of ad hoc explanation will force the kind of discriminative thinking you want to develop.

C_3 is highs and lows in feelings or activities. This should be a sacrosanct element of your diet diary because absolute freedom to write without "intimate" editing is crucial (13.40). Every day has its highlights and lowlights. Learn to identify at least one peak or trough for the sake of color. Strictly black and white characterization of existence implies depression. Embarking on the diet road means experiencing the transition to surrealistic color (fig. 8). Chapter 13 concerns a plethora of mixed emotions associated with errant thinking.

C_4 is exercises actually done. If you've done no exercises then write "none." It's surprising how satisfying it is to record this work that was done strictly for yourself. Exercise on the job doesn't count because it's already figured in to your current weight (chpt. 5).

C_5 is a precise number representing your final level of hunger just before sleep. Look back on "☉♉" with scrutiny. If you ate too much, resolve to eat less the next day. If you didn't get enough good food, have a small snack and go to bed (fig. 7). Marked hunger at others times is C_3 material. Against this spirit of wanting you'll do well to count your tender mercies, those aspects of your life that are good now.

Daily Waltz

Table 5

Final Hunger Level Quantitation

-3 = starved (not appropriate, eat, 13.308)

-2 = "starved" (have a light fruit snack)

-1 = "little bit hungry" (ideally)

0 = "not hungry" (what victories missed?)

+1 = "full" (too much this evening?)

+2 = "stuffed" (an extensive C2 required)

Whether this diet diary is kept strictly for yourself or you plan to seek mentor assistance depends on your personal inclination (chpt. 12). Do you usually prefer to deal with questions and problems alone? Certainly you must select your mentor with great care (13.54). The artistic manipulation of your body via enhanced control over intimate forces is not a process you should indiscriminately share.

Basically, you write to track the way your hands move through time and space. Developing such a record helps maintain the patient attitude and long-view so necessary to successful dieting. Music makes long trips more tolerable. An expert musician or mechanic can not teach delicate techniques by *mere talking to* a novice.

Hands on instructive experience with an actual model is necessary for learning. Tennis, swimming, or golf pros use video recordings of their students to teach advanced skills and visualize problems for correction (chpt. 6). Special motion cameras have taught much about the slow processes of flowering plants (chpt. 8). Final shoot-outs in popular T.V. detective series are often done in slow-motion. Climaxes of concerts, though they occur fast, actually are the result of very slow, painstaking practice and learning over quality time (chpt. 9; fig. 13).

The one-two-three daily diet **cadence** provides the rhythmic background onto which you can sketch in your own intrinsic melody line in life. Eventually, successively higher orders of rhythm can be developed until your vital sign of weight behaves like your other vital signs—automatically pitched at an optimal level for you. Life's colored mirrors variegate your performance setting—like *dancing in a dream*.

♀?♀ and ♀♀ develop the interface of your light and dark aspects of being. Dreams afford direct access to your subconscious. The dark side should be approached cautiously (13.200). The positive components of the dark side contain valuable elements such as your childhood sense of imagination and your adult "will to power." The *climax* of dieting essentially occurs in this turbulent twilight zone.

CHAPTER 12
MENTOR

A good mentor *candidly* orchestrates, catalyzes, and escorts the dieter by providing a personalized medium in which to acquire the diet hand skill (fig. 1). Superstition flourishes between the cavernous cracks of technological achievement (e.g. 13th floor of skyscrapers?). Sorcery exists just beyond the limits of rational knowledge; Merlin still inhabits modern vestiges of medieval forests and can enlist the best of human spirit to battle contemporary evil (figs. 8-10).

Mentors help the dieter develop the "mind's eye." Ubiquitous seducers obfuscate the Good via deceptions (poems 5, 6). Diet progress occurs best within the context of good vision, not muddy thought (chpts. 6, 13). Dieters need to know when and where not to look as well...

> When the mythical hero performed great feats for the King of the Underworld to earn the right to reclaim his beautiful lover (who'd been bitten by a poisonous snake in the garden due to a jealous god) he was told, "Take her hand and go hither up this tunnel toward the light of the living world, but do not look at her during this journey or she will be lost to you forever."
>
> And he clasped tight her hand and did as he was bid joyfully, until, near the end, she screamed and he looked back inadvertently—and she was immediately torn from him and sucked into the depths of oblivion ... (fig. 2δ)

When the modern playwright willed himself back in time 50 years in pursuit of an exquisite actress, he persevered in courtship and finally consummated his timeless love (frg. 1). They played together in the joyous afterglow of their union until he reached into his vest pocket, brought out a neglected modern trinket; she screamed as he gazed upon it and was tornadoed back to the future alone: the magical spell shattered (13.64).

Mentors listen to the dieter's questions and answer with an array of germane knowledge. A customized blend of nutrition, medicine, history, literature, philosophy, and common sense promote *self-realization* through a frank exchange of ideas and constructive rituals (chpt. 11). A mentor can do little with 'burned out' material or the disingenuous pretender (13.303).

The mentor relates more to spiritual identity than social faces. For women, focus is often on figure improvement notwithstanding the wife/mother/employee services that tend to dominate living. For men, appealing to latent powers of sensitivity or masculine pride in body form prompts the quest for a diet victory. Of course, qualities so intermingle between the sexes that each person must be considered individually; yet both men and woman absolutely share the common physiologic health benefits of eating intelligently, eliminating deleterious FAT (chpt. 3).

Some carefully selected diet pills may occasionally be warranted to help a dieter get started along the road particularly if fat genes exist or there have been many diet failures (figs. 3, 11, initial hump of 13; 13.307). Diuretics can aid removal of excess salt and water if swelling or hypertension is a problem. Physician mentors may elect to use some diet medications so long as the purpose is clear and the follow-up adequate. Frequently other medications such as anti-hypertensives or anti-sugar pills can be scaled down or eliminated completely as major amounts of FAT come off. *New skills, not pills, are the sine qua non of star dieting.*

The most important job of the mentor is to inspire a **leap of faith** predicated upon the original diet impulse (fig. 1). Diet adventure can be exciting but definitely has its dark moments (13.200). Christian cosmology predicts entry into the bright heavens follows a life of ethical behavior, yet such behavior may well entail a deliberate choice of pain over devilish pleasure or worldly gain (tbl. 2; fig. 12).

You do not want the untenable position of trying to avoid all positive pain (chpt. 5; 13.202). Dieting is a moral purgatory replete with mild pain and cast within your own will. A mentor must respect the designs of your being as it labors against universally destructive forces towards a delicate new state (13.54). As your soul proceeds to move through time and space in the sense of crusade, so arises the universal trace of your destiny (e.g. mG). The good mentor delineates the cacophony of personal demons threatening your diet course and suggests specific *strategies* for overcoming dietbusters.

Part II
COUNTERPOINTS

CHAPTER 13
DIETBUSTERS

Introduction 13.00

Demons lurk in the sinister shadows of the darkened path of your diet destiny. The poor light makes discerning the right way perilously difficult. Fierce roars, piercing howls, and ominous rattles knife through the eerie stretches of abject solitude (fig. 8). Your diet hopes hinge on a silver, starlight beam that guides you through the mire...

Fragment 2

Finale

And would you dream that I implore	(☉)
Upon my knees forever more:	(13.310)
Turn back your time to virgin lust	(chpt.9)
Do not burn out to spiteful dust	(13.41)
Strip naked now, be spirit free	(☹☹☹)
Without defense, deceit, or fee	(☉☹)
Like moon, night sky my dreams of thee..	(☹☹)
Your love was fleeting, hardly said	(13.303)
My love persists though nearly dead	(chpt.14)
It hangs by silver, starlight thread...	(chpt.12)

The high stress of dieting will *amplify* difficult themes in your life, especially love issues. Many a diet ship launches in close proximity to divorce, or, more subtly, because of cracks in the marriage foundation—fading interest (or passion) by one party (fig. 11). Conflicts about money usually have a worse effect on the state of marriage than issues of faith (13.64).

Some regression is natural before you can move forward. The foregoing distinctions between the three internal and the three external resistances blur in the misty field of actual battle. Generally, strict adherence to doing and recording the 15 min./day daily waltz rituals plus *selective* mentor inputs will suffice to vanquish each dietbuster (chpt. 11; fig. 9). The test of time yields truth, especially if you steadily face reality with consistent honesty.

Exquisitely armed with truth and honest will, how can you not do what you want with your own hands? You're not a baby anymore. *Variegated* formulations of adult dietbusters resist individually: desire, fear, specious reasoning, intimates, non intimates, et al. (fig. 10). The fun part of dieting combines heroic detective work with evolving beauty—a prescription for an adventure story with a happy ending.

Desires 13.10

"I want it all: now!," "I do what I want," "I get what I want!" are primitive extensions of healthy positivism: "I can do it!" Selfish over-applications of such principles re sex, business, or politics have indeed yielded some spectacular results historically: empires created and destroyed, promiscuous lustings followed by V.D., a vast trail of resultant human misery. Often crashing health ends these great sagas of egocentricity.

The high point of star dieting is **tempered** desire, i.e. maximization of all pleasures at the lowest possible final cost. What good is an interminable succession of fleeting pleasures in seductive foods if over-indulgence yields a despicable figure and plummeting self-esteem? How can values be shifted to smartly acquire *as much as you care to have?*

Dietbusters

Scale Junky 13.11

You *bunny-hop* on and off the scales every day, and look for instant results with each diet effort. Anxious to get it over with as soon as possible (i.e. get back to some serious enjoyment of food), you strip absolutely naked and try mild upward self-levitation when gingerly stepping upon the scales. If you've lost a fraction of a pound since yesterday you feel elated. If you've gained notwithstanding some hunger-suffering, you mope the rest of the day.

Calm yourself. Remember hares win battles, not wars (chpt. 10; fig. 13). Owners of stock have the same problem if they fret over every daily change in the price per share. Daily weighing spurs meaningless emotional swings which can easily disassemble a diet by frantic disequilibrium (13.207). Dieting stirs your physiologic soup and heats up your diurnal variations in water content, hormone activity, and bowel habits. In short, daily weights ironically distract from dieting: don't do it.

Enjoy the *drama* of weekly weighing. Consecutive weekly weights over one year generate extremely valuable feedback numbers especially when faithfully recorded (13.313). Look upon the entire week as one meal in relation to your net gain or loss. Your sense of time will expand (chpt. 9). Though the older or incapacitated should lose slower, 5-10 lbs. a month is a fine rule-of-thumb rate. The diet itself should be savored, not wolfed down.

Routine Seductions 13.12

You know what gets to you: savory sausage for weekend breakfast, ice cream when you're hot, hot chocolate when you're cold, salted popcorn with the VCR big movie, a rich wedge of pie for the big-talking business lunch, a cigarette after a fine meal, coffee with sugar and cream to start a working day, your favorite candy bar late in the day for energy, alcohol after work, a bread derivative with every meal, some fatty red meat every day.

Your **'passion differential'** is as specific as your fingerprint (fig. 1). Setting and timing for your urges are patterned. These routine seductions may have pounded your past diets to a pulp; you can't seem to escape the gravitational pull of them. The notion of heavenly orbit within your goal range seems more and more implausible.

Your strategic edge in routine seductions is precise knowledge of the enemy gleaned from analysis of your diet diary. Prepare a defense. Learn to *anticipate* and ignore ambush cues (13.43). *Divert* your hands from cookie to fresh fruit, or smoke a carrot instead of a cigarette—you'd look no more ridiculous. *Wait out* some regular urges. Each finite wave of hunger arrows subsides (figs. 10, 12). *Blunt* specific seductions—if the smell of freshly cooked bacon seems irresistible just take a wiff of ammonia in cleanser.

If you do suffer a defeat, then add some more positive pain to the next exercise session to *punish* yourself (chpt. 5). Literally account for all defeats (C_2). *Look* for the dark truth about your dietbusters beyond the obvious.

Special Seductions 13.13

You "go crazy" and "pig out" when presented with a special banquet of delicious food (fig. 12). You pass by routine seductions admirably and start losing some "serious weight" until the siren calls of special seductions wreck your diet ship (13.12; fig. 11).

That wild office party, the sweet smile of your grandchild over her birthday cake, the annual vacation, the permissive spirit of your favorite holiday, or any unusual, *intoxicating* sense of extraordinary times can lull you to sleep at the helm—so that you wake up to discover the currents have swept you irreversibly off course or you're drowning in 'serial sin' (fig. 10).

Immediate assistance comes from strict adherence to the diet *diary format*: writing all you eat and drink as soon as possible tends to sober the soul, break the mystique of the moment. Certainly, that nightly review of defeats will temper your next performance. Often the evening result of a day of high-living "junk food" is malaise, particularly beyond youth, when gastrointestinal, enzymatic capacity to digest a fattening bolus diminishes.

Do you buy something simply because you come across a sale of it? Do you habitually overextend yourself with credit card currency? Your approach to special seductions should be dependent on actual earnings. Below your goal weight you may welcome exotic seductions and enjoy the full gamut of special treats. Above your 'trigger weight' you must regretably pass the sweets but enjoy the atmosphere nevertheless (chpt. 15).

Credit card mentality—"buy now, pay later"—can lead to massive deficits, obesity. Business expansion based on sound fundamentals deserve credit, but wild gaining and losing (weight or money) disturbs your peace of mind per se.

After all, money is only paper articles of *faith* in the government (13.64). Yet if the economy crashes it's not the same as your crashing into the emergency room because of the effects of rampant obesity. The pages of your diet diary constitute the venture capital required to create your desired state.

Faith and money flow together, especially in special situations. Invest in yourself. Do your diet diary faithfully. Eventually, star dieting actually enhances your enjoyment of saying "yes!" to special seductions (when below your trigger weight) because you know all those "no's" of the dieting process mean that you've truly earned it.

Addictions 13.14

Every day you obsessively indulge in your "number one" pleasure. You think you ought to be able to control your desires for this deleterious item yet you consistently have proven that you can not. Your mind can twist into pretzels justifying your habit; but in your heart you feel like a **prisoner** of fattening passion. Your addiction affords a sickening glaze over life or a phony "high" (fig. 6). You hate yourself for what you want to do every day yet indignantly attack anyone that suggests you need to "get a hold of yourself."

No special calling is required to reach for your favorite addiction—any reason, any time, is special enough (13.13). You're a closet fanatic, a lush. You prefer to get your daily fix inconspicuously. You're clever about masking the addiction, even from yourself, if you can.

Your potential list of addictions is quite diverse. Every day you simply must have some form of your favorite passion. Processed sugar comes in so many forms it's easy to disguise your ravenous desire for it. Pop can have sugar or salt or addictive flavorings to great excess. Many smokers freely acknowledge their ravenous dependence because the odors, raspy voice, chronic cough, and actual consumption are impossible to hide (whereas the etiology of obesity is much "cleaner"). Alcoholics also have trouble hiding—slurred speech, wild behavioral swings, staggering gait, and diminished performance as well as their characteristic odors. The *fact* of obesity is usually obvious; the *mechanism* of obesity can be quite elusive.

Intimates tend to know the truth about the addicts with whom they live. When pressed, addicts claim to everyone that their (chemical) dependency has such overwhelming force that they are quite justified in their failures to escape.

Many addictions initiate during the turmoil of late teenage years. Wrong forks can become personal traditions or prisons with *no apparent exit* (fig. 5). Trying to break out causes hysterical withdrawal symptoms. The addiction is a *queer security blanket* upon which other disparate insecurities can be heaped indefinitely. After awhile, letting go may evoke dark fear akin to the basic fear of falling or being hurt (13.200). The addict does not want to tumble into a den of personal ghosts, tremors, weakness, and incessant nightmares.

Taking a wrong *sexual fork* can precipitate an overwhelming series of events: teenage pregnancy, frantic wedding, desperate follow-up pregnancies, onset of anxious overeating, divorce, unmasking of the original error, some self-defeating rebound relationships, then the sorrowful realization that aging, fatness, and depression have become habitual fixtures of life along with an addiction.

Or, as a teenager you become acquainted with parents whose ways of parenting differ dramatically from those of your own parents. Suddenly one or both of your parents don't measure up to your pristine ideals. The meanness of one parent in particular upsets you; even though that parent also smokes and hypocritically insists that you shouldn't smoke, you begin smoking because it calms your nerves and looks "grown-up". So your evolving *love-hate* relationship has the contradictory elements of emulation and rebellion through addiction (13.204). You're intense, you see flaws and contradictions everywhere, you seize upon a muddled assortment of declarations, and imprint some bad habits that might imprison you for life.

The protean etiologies of various addictions are innumerable (fig. 10). Often the very complex final forms of these addictions defy elucidation or direct cure. Certain foods, cigarettes, alcohol, or drugs can come to be a form of *intractable worship* (13.203). Interminable psychiatric probing can become addictive itself. Similarly, psychological "sessions" tend to prove fruitless. Addictive personalities transfer obsessions with lightning ease, just so they can escape facing dark realities (fig. 4; 13.200). Actually, the value to the addict of avoiding harsh truth rivals the "crutch" value of the addictive chemical on a day to day basis. Fortunately, it often doesn't matter how the addiction started. Star dieters seek only the amount of insight necessary to attain a viable *working solution* to the addiction problem.

Overwhelming addictions need direct treatment, quite possibly physician prescribed medications or professional counseling. Mild addictions are amenable to less drastic, more likely to succeed techniques.

First, you must simply see for yourself what you're doing. There's so much variety in food formats, timing, and perception that you may not realize your addiction until unmasked by a block in diet progress (fig. 2). Second, don't 'overthink' (13.318). Battling your addiction can itself become a distractive addiction. Third, decide whether you prefer a "cold turkey" or "diminishing mass" approach to defeating your addiction.

Fourth, honestly track your progress or failure in your diet diary. The longer you do this the better your chances of making a meaningful change for the better. Fifth, have *faith in yourself*. Seek outside help only as a last resort. Usually the extraneous trappings of outsider meddling result in futile labeling, rehashing, and reshuffling of a deck already stacked against you (13.307).

Cogent visualization spurs self-help because you tend to do what's best for yourself when you clearly see what's in your best interests (chpt. 6). Identification of the superficial addiction comes about far more easily than dealing with the underlying cause for dependency. An addiction need not be entirely fathomed nor totally "cured," just managed optimally.

Distractive Seductions 13.15

Cathy really needed to lose 80 lbs. She'd been heavy and shy since puberty. Boys never paid much attention to her in school though she paid attention to them. She learned the harsh truths of life coming from social neglect in high school. Her friends were also "wallflowers." After high school she worked as a cashier in a department store.

Because of a tip from a fellow employee she began to star diet. Her weight dropped precipitously—down 55 lbs. in five short months. Suddenly her natural beauty became self-evident and several men became keenly interested in her. She bought new clothes, new make-up, and developed a fairly glamorous demeanor. She avidly learned new sexual hand skills (fig. 1.3).

Despite the vast improvement in her figure and terrific love life, deep down she still felt fat and insecure—as always ("emot" fig. 13). Moreover, she began to experience greater highs and lows in her feelings than ever before (C_a). Some of these new men expressed jealousy towards her dates with other men and the ensuing turmoils of sexual politics frightened her (13.205). She ate more; she was both happy and upset about her new life. She stopped her diet diary. She gradually gained back 13 lbs. (fig. 2☾); her diet fate is indeterminate.

Naturally, concentration on dieting wavers when the waters of life churn tumultuously (tbl. 1; fig. 10; 13.56). Just as the dark undercurrents of Christmas season spur acute depression, so do the relational changes of a major diet success warrant a *warning* (poems 4, 10).

Throughout history there are stories of precipitous rises to power followed by rapid falls due to administrative abuses of that new power. Or, more simply, consider how the new walking, skating, or driving skills can initially "set-up" the latent showoff for a crash, a hard lesson. The seductive trappings of new power in sexual politics can decimate the originally pure spirit of a diet resolve.

Re-resolutions of ¶?¶? help keep the diet focus on the self until a constitutional consolidation is completed (chpt. 15). Specific external problems must be dealt with on an ad hoc basis. Usually, courteous perseverance coupled with some distancing from bold new initiatives will improve chances of circumventing too many positive distractions along the diet path. Complete the diet before starting any elective projects.

Fears 13.200

Star dieting occurs in the twilight interface of light realities and dark potentialities. As a child, fear of creatures in the dark vanished when the lights were turned on and comforting people came, i.e. conventional security in sight. However, public spotlights are too garish to nicely illuminate an intimate process like fashioning ones naked curves irrespective of de facto social norms accepting obesity. Thus star dieting is 'X-rated,' inherently private, stripped of cultural sanction per se.

Turn on the spotlights after the goal weight is attained (chpt. 16). Embrace, instead of run from, imagination. Confidentiality especially helps the fearful accomplish diet goals. Will power and confidence can selectively be evoked out of the dark side. . .

Poem 5

Dark Resolution

I have a habit, quite obscene	(13.203)
Of foolish talk and open heart	(13.304)
So with one exception—my mentor, dean	(chpt.12)
I vow a year of silence lean:	(mG)
Black Shroud surround my earnest life	(13.200)
And help me meditate towards grace	(℗℗℗)
Express myself and what I feel	(C₃)
With timing right, perspective real.	(chpt.9)

Sleep dominates nearly one-third of existence. Even when awake, light behavior is dramatically influenced by the underside of consciousness, subconsciousness. Fear of dark, fear of aspects of the dark self can paralyze a dieter (☾). In certain types of specious reasoning key dark forces actually develop insidious control of light-oriented hand-motor neurons and fattening foods seem to be consumed via evil magic (fig 12; 13.300): *star dieting is reciprocal magic*.

The forest of figure 8 represents the dark wilderness each soul must face alone along the diet trail. Whether darkness is globally evil or not depends on your world view or Weltanschaunng. Dark matter, its being, may overwhelm light matter in terms of cosmic physics. Cosmology influences eating via faint astrological forces and aesthetic metaphysics (frag. 2; tbl. 2). Ethics is only the bright tip of an iceberg of dim hope drifting through indifferent currents of infinite space (poem 8).

More than hot desire, specious reasoning, or blatant interference from others, the fear of direct confrontation with the *personal specters doth chill the will of dieters*. Inner illumination (poem 6) fosters the best way to overcome such adversity, courageously.

Anxiety 13.201

You worry all the time. Headaches, back pain, stomach distress, insomnia, or weakness plague you constantly. You've taken all sorts of pills, worry about your health, yet get no relief. You also *fret* about money, your children, even the continued love of your spouse.

Your friends kindly pretend you're not getting fat and dumpy. You avoid wearing swimsuits in public pools and seek ambiguous clothes to hide your figure. You go to beauty salons weekly for your hair and nails yet you don't really feel the least bit beautiful.

You do less actual work yet seem far more tired than ever before in your life. Working, driving, shopping, and other routine chores are all fraught with concerns that leave you quite tired and hungry by evening (13.52).

You especially worry about your increasing fatness, so you eat more (13.300). Afterwards you're filled with guilt because you know you've only made things worse yet you can't seem to stop yourself when you get the urge for fattening products. Diet products and sweet snacks sit side by side in your pantry. You overeat not because of hunger, rather, you seek that temporary rush of pleasure you get from a wide variety of seductions (fig. 6).

Of course, you assuage your guilty consciousness by dieting regularly and you have first hand knowledge about why a large variety of diet techniques do not work (fig. 2B; 13.303, 13.320).

Neither anxiety nor happiness are amenable to direct action; they come about *indirectly*. Concentrate on the center of the wheel—yourself (fig. 1). Don't overrate prayer or strength outside yourself because in order to endure, the diet skill should be broached essentially alone (chpt. 15). Who else perceives your dark secrets so clearly? Successful dieting can be like flipping a magic switch that turns your entire life from quiet desperation to bright happiness (13.200; chpt. 16). The cornerstone of a new life should be yourself...

Poem 6

Waking

Finally, I turned within to see what would be
For it's inlook in life that in living I see
Makes all the difference—in peace or in tax
One thing matters most: that I wisely relax.

Freud predicted anxiety would be the chief problem of this century, echoing Wordsworth ("The World Is Too Much with Us"). The desultory character of modern living deeply disturbs many lives. Fattening foods do provide some respite, some semblance of steady satisfaction (fig. 6).

Besides the formal mechanism for dieting indicated in this book, here are some scattered suggestions for alleviating anxiety on a daily basis: 1) exercise within your limits while thinking about possible ways you might deal with specific problems (chpt. 5); 2) routinely get a body massage from an intimate; 3) read history for perspective (reading any good literature tends to calm the spirit); 4) write e_a cathartically in your diet diary; 5) actively pursue previously dormant personal interests that make you feel good; 6) take strategically planned brief mininaps during the day (in prayer or yoga sense of reaching for serenity within); 7) sip warm liquids to help fall asleep early at night; 8) listen to peaceful music without commercials (13.55).

Generally, optimistic focus on bettering your life through consistently *uplifting activity* alleviates anxiety (fig. 13). Though dieting superficially causes craving-driven hysteria, the net result will be fundamental peace within an improved naked being.

Pain 13.202

Your children dive right into the spring water, but you just toe in briefly—you'll wait till summer when it's nice and warm. You've come to prefer lukewarm showers to really invigorating hot or cold. You don't *exert* yourself anymore because you get so short of breath easily and because you feel so sore the next day.

Similarly, the quality of your work is tepid. You note that so-half productivity gets you the same paycheck as if you had made the extra effort to do a good job. You don't take the stairs when an elevator is available. You fantasize about winning a lottery or inheriting money but take no business initiatives to increase your fortunes. You never act on attainable dreams or ambitions.

You'd generally rather watch than do, buy than make, win than earn. So a T.V. diet gimmick that promises loss of weight and beauty without effort gets your rapt attention.

When diet hunger pain comes you guiltlessly eat or drink anything at hand to eradicate it (13.308). You're not anxious, you just diet with tepid zeal (13.201; fig. 2a). You've broadened the universal fear of negative pain to include positive pain as well (chpt. 5).

There's a progressively hotter bed of coals between your current and goal weights over which you must walk barefoot. To minimize the pain, briskly walk one straight path from start to finish (tbl. 1). Don't hop off just near the end (fig. 2ð). As a stone drops surely and swiftly to the bottom of a lake so should your spirit pursue your goal weight.

Prior to birth the fetus floats in warm liquid, all needs provided, a carefree existence. The rude awakening of birth mandates breathing, eating, etc. Fear of falling becomes a reality that discourages courageous leaps (fig.1). If the major goal of life is reapproximation of the luxury of a relatively painless, enclosed, warm, passive existence (e.g. to be rich and live at an exotic island resort), then dieting will indeed be difficult for such dreamers because a **daily tincture of pain** must be willfully embraced to succeed; this applies to any worthwhile way to structure time beyond conventional expectations (chpts. 1, 5, 9).

The will power required to overcome a wave of hunger pain is about equal to the courage to dive into a cool swimming pool or taking a cold shower. Surprisingly, many people develop such an extreme aversion to pain that they eschew even trivial forms.

Not only do pain thresholds differ widely among races of people, but a given individual can raise or lower their own tolerance levels (C_4, C_5). Star dieters seek to attain a moderate increase in their positive pain *tolerance* along with a greater *zest* for diving into life.

Intractability 13.203

You don't worry that much, nor does pain scare you (13.201, 13.202). You've basically lived each day similarly for many years. You're steady as a rock both at work and at home. The occasional vacation or crisis causes mild ripples which die out quickly. You note new things but make no special effort to pursue them.

You raise your children exactly the same way that you were raised and you're surprized when they seem to have interests unique to the family. At family reunions you're aware of gossip about the "black sheep" of the family yet don't really understand the sense of this deviant behavior.

You're annoyed your weight has drifted up even though you've appropriately eaten less as you've aged (figs. 2,3). You're not frantic about your FAT, just perturbed (13.318). You eat and drink the same kinds of foods your family has characteristically consumed for many generations. And you blend right in with the other FATS at family gatherings.

But you've never entirely accepted your FAT. You know it's not good for health and would prefer not to be so far overweight. You actually dieted a few times without noticeable effect (fig. 2λ). Perhaps your family is full of the "fat genes" that tend to make people fat irrespective of consumption (13.307).

Traditions indeed exert enormous influences on life and invariably involve food. Birthdays feature birthday cakes, Thanksgivings and Christmas incite great carbohydrate excesses, New Years triggers high ethanol consumption, Valentines and Halloween involve excessive candy, etc.

Most obesity arises from *fattening traditions* coupled with modern stresses. If the parents themselves liked bacon sandwiches, or rice, or gravy and biscuits, or pasta dishes, or alcohol, or some bread form with every meal, or special types of pies and cakes, then probably their children and their children's children will follow suit. Some may have "thin genes" or high metabolisms that protect them from obesity, but most will be at least moderately overweight, especially those that struggle with living.

Cultural traditions frequently associate big events with big carbohydrate excesses. Football means beer. Baseball connotes hot dogs. Parties imply ethanol. Picnics include sugar water and deserts. The protean associations of good times with specific fattening food patterns of consumption in families run throughout a year (fig.10; chpt.9; 13.51). It's quite a *trick* to escape the massive gravitational pull of all these fattening traditions (fig. 2 inverted; 13.47).

The most important point to grasp when you endeavor to change the status quo for yourself is the absence of luck in dieting (chpt. 1). You're interested in **discriminating** what features of traditions are valuable and which may be regarded as strictly optional. When you attend a birthday party you must show love and respect, no one should really care whether or not you eat the birthday cake too. Distinguish between family fun and true communion.

When you loosen your grip on any aspect of family tradition you'll have to face the resistances of other family members to your initiative as well as your own fear of falling into the void of anarchy (fig. 1; chpt. 14). Often a major *leap of faith* must be made to significantly break with undesirable aspects of the family status quo for appropriate behavior at key times. Moreover, besides new values, you'll have to develop an ad hoc etiquette to smooth out ripples your deviant actions may cause.

"Status quo" implies considerable political force. Many traditions enrich human lives immeasurably. If, however, you feel trapped in a FAT prison promoted by family habits that you can do without, then have the courage to accomplish a minor revolution uniquely (tbl. 1). *Respect* major traditions but *pass* on fattening embellishments: the sky won't fall.

Familial Fear 13.204

You're frantically afraid you're getting to look like some of your FAT blood relatives. Even as a child you sensed that you didn't want to resemble a particularly obnoxious FAT uncle or aunt. You might remember how FAT grandma or grandpa turned ashen, panted for breath, and spit out that horrible stuff one time they tried to play with you in the park; from then on they just sat on the bench and smoked while you played with other children.

After you'd reached teenage years you became aware how FAT your parents were; it embarrassed you. You knew you were never going to be FAT yourself, like your sister or brother had become. Yet now you're *horrified* to admit that FAT has unmistakably gained a foothold on your naked body (fig. 1). Even worse, you once dieted nearly all the way to your goal weight only to gain it all back, plus more FAT (fig. 2ô). Or, now that you're approaching the age at which your FAT parent died, your acceptance of FAT for yourself wavers: you fear your imminent death (13.203).

Unlike those that basically accepted the family status quo you secretly resisted getting fat all along; your notion didn't work satisfactorily because your different values were not backed up by *new experiential skills*. So you succumbed to the fattening flow of culture.

The defiant "no" you developed as a child when given instructions not to play as you intended to play may be usefully brought out of mothball status. A firm "no, thank you" should deflect the force of a FAT relation's insistence that you follow in their FAT path rather than your own (fig. 8). You have a right to establish some good traditions yourself.

Jealousy 13.205

You've been slowly getting heavier ever since you were married, especially after pregnancy. Your husband seems to be gone more and more for business or pleasure. You're jealous his attention is elsewhere; he's jealous of other men. You get

Dietbusters

lonely and depressed when he is gone: that's why you eat more than you know you should (13.41). Sometimes when he comes home he flies into a rage over nothing; moreover, despite fleeting "good times," his overall interest in satisfying you sexually has plummeted.

Every time you lose weight your former beauty returns and even men in the church choir pay too much attention to you. Your "friends" circulate vicious rumors about your intentions towards their husbands (13.45, 13.47). When these false rumors reach your husband, his unjustified suspicions are inflamed. You try harder yet your self-esteem is driven lower (13.319).

Your spouse is no longer a romantic suitor; he now concentrates on the practical profits out of your marriage: sex his way, catered meals, extra money because of your sacrifices, plus free care of his children. The passion that seemed like everything in the beginning of your relationship is now weak. You get fatter while he oogles all the young, slender beauties he sees.

Of course, he regards a precipitous rise in your level of femininity with alarm, especially as you penetrate the primary fat zone (tbl. 1). You fear his jealous wrath and he fears the challenge of keeping pace with your evolving to a level of sophisticated beauty much higher than the level on your wedding day. He senses his own subtle declines in physical appearance (intrinsic jealousy). The "beer belly" he jokes about actually disturbs his masculinity. He can no longer keep up with his own sons in sports (extrinsic jealousy).

The *security* of the status quo of a marriage will be markedly threatened if one party dramatically rises in self-esteem while the other is left far behind. Resistance to changes in the status quo, on the other hand, protects the static party from a premature adjustment to a bogus foray.

Most husbands profess love irrespective of the wife's level of fat. Most husbands do not significantly assist a major diet by their partner (13.44). About 10% of husbands encourage outright, 70% give mixed signals, 20% show considerable jealousy; these numbers apply to a variety of other intimate associations.

The jealous groups require a measure of reassurance that your dieting will not affect your feelings for them; unless it does.

Obviously, if you suddenly reverse a decade or two of getting FAT then the status quo will have to change both privately and socially when you succeed (13.203). A major component of the "emotion" wagon will be smoothing over the variety of changes ensuing at your goal weight (fig. 13).

Provincial, malicious politics are everywhere, so just weather the squalls your enhanced beauty generates. Many diets are wrecked by jealous recrimination (fig. 11). More than one diet diary has been burned. Life for all your relations will just have to shift a bit as you take a little more personal time (chpt. 9). Eventually, everyone will adjust and the new status quo will be better for all.

Sexuality 13.206

As a teenager you were intensely interested in sex. After marriage the bedroom fire waned. "And they lived happily ever after" gave way to bills, children, tedium, a cacophony of practical concerns: you now overeat for compensatory pleasure (fig. 6).

You say that "you don't have time" to briefly caress yourself and write a few notes in your diet diary in the morning because from the moment you get up you chase behind the carrot of interminable chores—like a donkey doomed to a life of incessant labor (♀?♀; 13.301, 13.319).

Actually, by refusing to do your morning ritual (before you get caught in a network of practical chores) you're revealing your preference for an adorned, social self over a naked, private self. You're still interested in sex but engage far more in eating for direct pleasure; it's easier. Gossip, romance novels, and "soaps" dominate your parasexual thoughts; such vicarious glamor and sex does not involve *risk* on your part.

You have come to fear expression of your own sexuality for some reason, probably as it relates to an intimate. You can not remember the last time you actually explored a new sexual technique in your bed. You flatly deny the relevance of sex or glamor to your diet. You say you just want to lose weight for health.

Serious dieting may well entail squarely facing an old sexual fork in the road (fig. 5). Unsolved, intimate problems such as a crack in the crystal of your marriage may well be quite relevant since FAT pours through such openings (13.00).

For example, marriages launched by teenage pregnancy often involve two partners lacking in self-confidence, neither having spent much time out in the "real world" away from parents. As the babies arrive an insecure marriage drives further into trouble. Lust vanishes in the face of overwhelming responsibilities.

One or both spouses sublimate sexuality to concentrate on earning money or performing domestic tasks in such a way as to cope with a desperate situation; or they simply grow apart. Typically the husband will be the one who runs away rather than try and work things out. Typically the wife most directly sublimates sexuality for the sake of reducing confrontation.

Resistance to caressing the naked body for the sake of artistic acquaintance with the *undeniably naked subject* of the diet often stems from a fear of broaching troublesome sexual topics directly (♀?♀); if there exists strong sexual underpinnings to the original diet resolution, then this *gentle self-confrontation* evokes the pertinent history of sexual politics at some point (chpt. 8).

An independent resolution to diet is divorced from jealous spouse interference (chpt. 2). Theoretically, by enhancing the sexual implications of your figure your spouse should only derive benefit—heightened sexuality and social appreciation (13.40). Practically, many direct resistances to increasing your sexual appeal may exist even if your original intent was not overtly sexual (13.205).

Fear of the "other woman" or the effect of other spheres of sexuality may either stimulate overeating or spur a diet resolution. Just as an juvenile error in the steering skill may lead to a crash so might a deviation in sexuality lead to divorce (fig. 1). **Irrationality** underlies most sexual politics ("all is fair in love and war," 13.307). Primate territoriality and the imagined demarcations of sexual privilege have much in common. Since sexual fears can have no rational basis, management does not require reason.

When sexual fear causes regressive behavior, then food becomes the equivalent of the toys of childhood. Obese people frequently display enormous interests in the art of cooking; they develop a keen sense of "playing" with food for fun; they talk about delicious food interminably. Their sexual imaginations lie dormant while their minds fill with details about food productions and consumptions.

Sexism dominates fundamental identity ("Is it a boy or a girl?") as well as toy distinctions. Boys get guns, girls get dolls; moreover, that's what they want. Flight into regressive food sexuality doesn't really help the fear of sex, though it can *mask* the fear indefinitely. Sexism affects dieting too. Women have a strong subculture supporting dieting yet are more likely to be maligned while dieting (13.205). Women usually know more about food options and are more sensitive to what they're eating. Men tend to drift in dieting yet have a stronger sense of direct association of sport and weight control.

The combination of fear of abject sexuality and specious reasoning usually indicates intractable burnout. Resolving sexual fears associated with dieting is a vast topic beyond the scope of this book. Suspend doubt and proceed with the diet diary in good faith. Seek out a good mentor (chpt.12). Each case must be dealt with on an individual basis because so many disparate forces collide irrationally, hence, algorithms are effete.

Highs & Lows in Feelings 13.207

You say you just "don't have the will power" but your diets actually fail because you are swamped by highs or lows in feelings (13.308; $C_{\mathring{a}}$). The closer you get to your goal weight the more violent the waters become (tbl. 1; fig. 11). The *buffeting* arises as common emotional swings are amplified during the intrinsic stress of dieting.

Though your spouse has never been particularly jealous before, now he perversely presses you to quit, to "prove" your devotion (13.205, 13.206). You get ravenously hungry or retain water going into your period (fig. 4). Living off FAT cells as much as possible has made you quite irritable towards everybody (chpt. 3). You display hair-trigger anger at your children's antics, husband's idiosyncrasies, or society's hypocrisies (13.40). You want the world to stop for awhile till you get your weight right again (13.55). "Good times" rock your diet vessel too (chpt. 9).

Poem 7

Nature's Parts

Darting here, darting there	(13.301)
The particles seem not to care	(13.307)
A system gained, a system lost	(13.311)
On seas of change my fate is tossed	(13.309)

Religious completion of a *sacrosanct* diet diary ballasts the ship through the final squalls. Basic being moves not with respect to the superficial gales of hectic modern living, but rather the great mass of value moving through dark rivers of time. The mentor should assist subtle value shifts into the right channels (chpt. 12; fig. 5).

Near the end of any great roller coaster ride are a series of scary highs and lows leading to a *grand climax*, a **'kinesthetic gestalt'** (fig. 13). Initiating the star diet constitutes the first "leap of faith," boarding (fig. 1). Relax and experience subsequent highs and lows since jumping out near the end leads to no good (fig. 2ბ; poem 4). Besides, you can not jump off the world; and it will not stop for you.

Attitude most determines resolution outcomes (chpt. 2). While feelings are the cutting edge of personality, patterns of reactions to feelings dominate *action*. Will power to do the proper actions of dieting can be derived from marshaling reactive forces into effective hand movement via attitude (fig. 1).

Thus, the high turbulences of dieting stem from shifts brought about by value tremors in relation to dynamic evolution of personality. A scathingly honest diet diary proves to be an invaluable tool for visualizing these abstractions (chpt. 6). The star dieter seeks *to master reactions to highs and lows in feeling through insight.*

Protean Resistances 13.208

As you lose more weight you are overwhelmed by the diversity of obstacles that arise against continued progress (fig. 10). Though you do not relish a dogfight, the internal battles that constitute a diet civil war comes with the hostile terrain (chpt. 10; fig. 8).

Concentrating on weight alone doesn't help (13.11). Dealing with protean resistances is like learning to *juggle* many parameters. First, concentrate on one relevant object at hand. Second, progressively increase the number of items you can manage at one time. Sketch the setting and the emotional context of the two or three major diet seductions of each day (C_1, C_2). Third, acquire a sense of the "big picture" so that you're automatically doing many small things right with respect to the overall effect you want (13.207; C_3). Many dieters completely lose sight of their diet because the complexity of modern living distracts them from the task at hand.

If you can juggle red objects you can usually also juggle blue ones (even of quite different sizes, shapes, and weights). Though any major diet will entail several fat zones and many diverse antagonistic feelings, it is possible to calmly master your weight via your diet diary.

Seek help if you do not clearly see your archetypal dietbuster (chpt. 6). You can not possibly handle a swarm of dietbusters near the end if you miss the main one in the beginning (fig. 9). It is quite disturbing to think you're in control, because you've lost some weight, only to be swamped by an array of problems you do not fathom.

Gauntness & Fat Distribution 13.209

One slashing comment from a friend can pique a torrent of concern about the point of dieting whatsoever (13.45). Fear of exacerbating facial aging due to gauntness can spook a dieter. When bloated facial FAT comes off relatively early in a diet then wrinkles may well become more apparent.

Movie stars are often better known at 40 years old than at 20 years old; yet they are considered very beautiful despite the existence of more wrinkles. Wrinkles also have a connotation of character and wisdom. So the fact that more wrinkles appear as a face becomes deflated of FAT is not necessarily a signal to abandon ship (fig. 11). Moreover the manifest beauty of a more youthful figure plus the enhanced inner spirit of the successful dieter nicely compensates for a tincture of gauntness in the face.

Nevertheless, women that lose FAT easily in the face should take care to lose weight slowly and not get caught in cycles of dieting often (13.310). Dieting is an attempt to rapidly reverse deteriorations set off by aging (fig. 3). So dieting can be viewed as a harsh physiologic stress against the tide out (with the "wave" in, chpt. 1). Stress tends to show in the face in general.

Ideal fat distributions in a mature woman vary according to the *aesthetic whims* of the culture. The hips, breasts, stomach, thighs, legs, and face have fat cells with different affinities for a given globule of blood fat. Different fat cells metabolize a given globule at slightly different rates as well (chpt. 3).

Your relative fat distributions vary in different zones with the specificity of your fingerprint (fig. 1; tbl. 1). If you want big breasts rather than big thighs then you may well be frustrating yourself for nothing (13.307). You may want to tolerate a little FAT in the hips to keep your breasts acceptably big. **Compromise** permeates body politics, a reasonably well-adjusted person, stable state (13.64). Virtually everyone has trivial physical parameters about themselves that they would prefer to alter.

Elective plastic surgery, even when technically successful, often fails because the real problem is insecurity rather than wrinkles or fat distribution. It's often better to cut out poor values and fashion in better ones than tinker with nature.

Concentrate on looking as good as you can without overthinking (13.321, 13.323). Those people that consistently overthink trivialities are not happy at any weight, nor any time. The appropriate principle of makeup and clothes is to highlight your best features. Fears about gauntness and fat distribution should be tactfully ignored.

Choking 13.210

You break into tears for no apparent reason just as you near your diet goal. You can't believe you've come so far only to discover that really deep down you never believed you'd win. Now you wonder what you'll do next. How will you keep FAT from returning? Can you handle all this extra attention you receive indefinitely?

The diet hand-skill spectrum merges laterally into the performance levels of individualistic sports; only the parameters of the game differ somewhat. Watch virtually any major tennis tournament and you'll see two world-class players of relatively equal technical ability square off (you can not discern who'll win on the basis of the warm-up). Yet the champion will nearly always win in the end.

Even if the winner has a slight lead and actually a numerical chance to win, he'll suddenly execute an unforced error, or get stunningly passed at the net by the champion on a *crucial point* that effectively decides the match; thereafter the champion rises to peak form while the winner wilts to near tears.

Every year a major golf tournament ends the same way—a novice winner of minor tournaments plays over his head and has a short putt on the last hole to win, yet lips out of the cup. Or the champion makes a series of fantastic shots to come from nowhere to force a playoff. Then the champion who has kept himself quietly in range of the leader eliminates his competition quickly in "sudden death." Just another routine tournament win for the champion, and another "rabbit" fades back into the pack for the rest of the season (fig. 13).

If, on the other hand, the "rabbit" hits a lucky shot to win, it's surprising news. Tis *aging* that eventually brings most champions down (frag. 3). Over twenty years old in swimming, thirty in tennis, forty in chess, fifty in golf—they just can't keep up with the emerging swell of youthful talent nor the ravages of time (13.209). When an aging champion wins, there's a flare of semi-nostalgic reporting, it's as if the dream of a fountain of youth could be vicariously realized (frag. 2).

After surviving a gauntlet of dietbusters and losing 90% of your excess FAT, you don't expect another major hurdle (13.322, 13.55). The critical distinction between a temporary diet winner and an enduring diet champion briefly appears small, but is actually great (fig. 2δ,ϵ). Essentially, *a second leap of faith* is required to make this climatic transition from winner to champion. The personality of the player in individual sports (mock war games) rather than the genius of the coach sets general outcome in nonteam sports (chpt. 2).

The romantic theme of dieting for glamor includes its warring elements too (chpt. 10; fig. 12). Sexual politics revolves around pleasure as perceived by territorial candidates (fig. 6). Often very major forks in the road of life are steered through according to very subtle yet fundamental distinctions in the caliber of performance within the competitive field of courtship (figs. 1, 5).

The champion deals decisively with the major seductions challenging ultimate victory or defeat. The champion steers into situations where there exists a winning response irrespective of the opponent's move.

The winner does great in minor combat, but chokes when it really counts. The lure of quitting (running from the stress of continuing the big game of dieting) often couples with the prospect of cheap, immediate pleasure (consuming some delicious deviation, thereby attaining sweet respite, fig. 6) to terminate resolve at the crucial point (resume "drifting," fig. 2). In contrast, *superior strategy and execution at critical moments are hallmarks of the champion* (fig. 13).

"Is that all?" 13.211

You ask me, "what's next?" This unfortunately fortunate question arises when you actually get exactly what you've wanted for a long time: high, safe, and stable at your goal weight, emotionally beyond "choking" (13.210; figs. 11, 13).

That odd fear of success of the winner gives way to glory (fleetingly) and then the challenge of pursuing *another dream* (chpt. 16); sometimes a void arises between the latter two stages (chpt. 14). This queer, desolate emptiness may provoke sarcastic questioning, even wild behavior. Before moving on to a fresh endeavor you may ironically glimpse the end of ends...

Fragment 3

Death

Destined to sense receding powers
And taste the pang of finite hours.

Multiple diet failures do tend to break the spirit and yield a sense of ennui, permanent burnout. The bored and listless line up in droves for each successive diet fad just prior to abandoning all hope (13.303).

A lamentable void typifies the "zone 4" intractables (tbl. 1). Like giant tumbleweeds on the plain of a vast desert, they tend to placidly languish in the sun; occasionally, they blow about according to desultory diet eddies, but wind-up rolling aimlessly upon a sea of shifting sand (FAT): pathetic "runaways" with neither point of origin nor even end-point mirage in view (13.322, 13.323).

In sharp contrast, the successful rarely taste more than a trace of despairing nihilism; they leave stoic dieting with vital currents in full force, relatively fearless, ready for the next adventure (chpt. 16). The answer to the question of this section is "no!" Learning γ grip raises the question of δ grip (fig. 1).

'Specious Reasoning' 13.300

Those people that routinely swear 'black is white' as it suits their self-interest in modern living will balk at the **scathing honesty** required to do a diet diary properly. Without the *grip* of the diet diary they can not proceed to learn subsequent *balance* and thereby ride to their goal weight by this method (chpt. 1).

The quandary of specious reasoning entails "overthought." The technique of utilizing "white lies" to considerable practical success over many years haunts the dieter. Like the boy that cried "wolf," credibility has been eroded, even for the self. The addictive habit of obfuscating the reality of your behavior in such a way as to present an image socially favorable to yourself will blur your own quality of inner vision over time (chpts. 6, 9).

Often the specious reasoner is intelligent; the cunning side of this intelligence can work directly against successful diet skill acquisition. The "high mind" simply won't admit what the hands are doing wrong as per the prompting of the "low mind" (figs. 1, 12); the answer to the indignant question, "Who did this!?" is to put the blame on someone else, "He did, certainly not me." After decades of dodging responsibility for misdeeds the internal distinction between *me* and *myself* becomes blurred. If a person overdoes self-serving deception externally, then as a dieter he tends towards self-deception internally.

Specious reasoners dominate diet talk both in casual conversations and public forums for dieters. Pretender diet experts proselytize one glittering inanity after another and persuade millions to follow their convoluted ways (13.54). Thus many specious reasoners acquire a cacophony of non sequiturs in which they place false hope.

Even when the specious reasoner has a burning desire to lose weight, an aberrant mechanism of diet thinking will twist their thoughts into **pretzeled prevarications**. The true mentor helps the dieter swing freely by *denuding* false notions. Enlightened travelers have a better chance of reaching their goal state (fig. 8).

"I'm too busy!" & "I forgot." 13.301

You plaintively say you're "too busy" to complete a diet diary or you "forgot" to make that critical entry of a fattening binge (13.315; fig. 12). You just don't feel like bothering to fuss with all that writing (13.317; chpt. 11). You're too busy making a living, doing your job as a good provider, sacrificing for others (13.319).

Or, you did your diet diary but forgot to bring it for mentor review because more practical matters demanded your full attention. Basically you argue that social obligations so swamp your consciousness that personal time is obliterated (chpt. 9). You simply grab what you can when you can conveniently. Whether it's "fast food" or just what you're served in business settings, you try to diet but fail because others essentially make you have fattening food (13.53).

The hysterical tempo of indiscriminate modern living warrants contempt and must be managed in the same sense as dieting rails against aging (figs. 2, 3). You can not change universal themes, but you can surf the tumultuous waves to shore smartly (chpt. 1; tbl. 1; fig. 11). Establishing one's rhythm of swimming is preferable to thrashing about frantically. The part names of this book allude to the establishment of optimal, autonomic weight rhythms that are more in tune with cosmic undulations of stars than pathetic, primate piddling.

You report that you're heroically caught in the swirling eddies of life such that your diets are doomed because of them; yet you *choose* to be caught as well. And how much time do you spend wastefully watching T.V., waiting for the next turn of the anxious wheel of fortune?

It takes less than 15 total minutes a day to do some exercises and complete all facets of the diet diary, about 1% of your total time available in a day. If you simply value your personal time above all, you'll be able to find 15 minutes somewhere amidst the turmoil. Use *ingenuity*.

Nothing's more convenient than an apple. Is it faster to travel, wait in line, pay, consume "fast food," and travel back for lunch or simply "brown bag" at a pleasant spot near your working place? Nutritious foods brought home after weekly shopping can be very conveniently carried to work. Even when traveling it's fairly easy to get ice, some kind of light container, some good food, and avoid all the trappings of "compulsory" fattening food. Besides it's far more expensive to pursue fattening foods at 3-5 times cost price to the buyer than taking the right fork (13.55; fig. 5).

Busy caregivers should know that they will get unfairly FAT if they eat right along with their metabolically more active children for the sake of convenience (13.307; fig.3). Yet even if those caregivers don't take a few moments to get something less fattening for themselves, it is often possible to have small portions and accomplish the same lower calorie intake ('principle of diminishing mass')

How much time does it take to prepare raisins, carrots, lean lunch meats, a little bread, fresh fruit, or water? Reach conveniently for what you *need* and *prefer* while dieting. Almost every menu has some nonfattening items. It takes no more time to order a simple hamburger rather than that Superburger and fries you usually get (mooch a few fries instead of ordering your own). Fortunately, diet water is usually available everywhere.

Let go of the myth that you're "too busy." You're undoubtedly not. If you *want*, then you can remember to diet properly for the sake of your naked figure and good health.

"It's impossible!" 13.302

You go significantly beyond the stance of the "busy body" or frenzied "white rabbit" (13.301). You declare that there's no way you can succeed at dieting because you've already tried everything and you just can't get around your recurrent problems. For example, your particular job as a salesman makes it impossible to diet because of interminable traveling, catered meetings, or total lack of practical support at home.

You're essentially *forced* to fail on your diets. You have no control over menus offered (13.55), the dictates of your business gatherings (13.53), nor what fattening foods get pushed in your face by well-intentioned family (you care about what these people think and wouldn't dream to possibly insult them or go against the fattening food flow of the moment, 13.47). Therefore, you're a captive of FAT now because of *others*. You bear little or no responsibility yourself because "God knows how you've tried" (poem 3).

Nonsense! You can devise a way to meet your needs and apply ad hoc etiquette to protect your diet (fig. 1). Though at least 5% of most menus include nonfattening choices, if you're truly limited to having only fattening food or an unacceptable nothing, then simply implement the diminishing mass principle—don't eat much. Lightly *taste* and *sample* enough to meet convenional expectations as well as your short-term energy needs.

Never reach for seconds. Smile sweetly and say "No thank you" when pushed to overeat the main course or have desert. Meet force with force (chpt. 9). If you're indignantly challenged to have more, then you don't have to account for your diet decisions, just nicely state how satisfied you are or vaguely refer to some unmentionable elimination problems, or something else equally unassailable.

Banish the pessimistic notion that your diet is doomed before you start. There's no luck in dieting (chpt. 1). Infinite varieties of personal resourcefulness exist. It's no one's business but your own what personal philosophy you pursue. Believe in yourself. Try.

'Pretender' 13.303

You make bountiful remarks about how hard you've dieted. You assert that you could write a book about dieting given all your monumental experience, knowledge, and suffering. God help anyone who directly suggests to you that you need to lose weight. Oh, how you've tried, how you're willing to try again just to prove what an especially difficult case you are (13.302). You say you'll give the star diet a chance to help you but frankly expect to fail from the start.

You're a consummate dietbuster yourself (fig. 9). Lord help the poor soul that enlists your advice and assistance in dieting (13.54). Attitude determines outcomes and yours is abysmal (chpt. 2). You go through each type of diet with a "chip on your shoulder." Soon you will announce that the star diet is inept and *cruise* off to another after some well-deserved binging. You've accumulated a long list of silly notions, pointed questions, and ways to attack the validity of any dieting program (pre-antidieter).

Insincerity torpedoes dieting (fig. 11). The pretender seems like a destroyer on the surface, a desperate swan underneath (*fear of burnout*). Pretenders huddle together for courage in "diet clubs" of one sort or another and frequently embark together on pointless derivations of fad dieting (chpt. 1). Deep down they're beginning to placidly accept total failure (tbl. 1). Moreover, the disingenuous dieter will fail on every diet program because aging can not be bluffed (fig. 3).

Life is beautiful. Start fresh and pursue your greatest share of wondrous existence. Let this diet be your first step to higher states of existence (fig. 8). Banish prior "knowledge" of the kind that alienates you from yourself. Reach not for bankrupt misconceptions. Seek faith with "fear and trembling."

Morning Faster 13.304

You pridefully declare that you "skip breakfast." Though your belly bursts with baleful blubber, you're not to blame because you nobly sacrifice that morning meal (except on weekends, when it's bacon or sausage as usual). Moreover, in abstractly discussing your dietary habits at the outset you highlight your virtues—avoiding sweets, salt, and other fattening tendencies plus the overall fact of "not eating that much." What a saint!?

But you're FAT! You talk like it shouldn't be so. You have an optimistic attitude about dieting yet you stay FAT. You've been FAT for a long time. You've been dieting on and off for a long time as well (fig. 2B, 2C). You don't understand what sinister forces thwart these diets of yours, especially since you've instigated the brilliant maneuver of "fasting" in the early day.

You omit the fact that you're not really hungry in the early day, so you've been sacrificing nothing all along. You distort the truth about your eating binges as the day wears on (13.52). You disregard all the snacking. You falsely believe that your regular diet deviations are paid for by these meaningless morning fasts. You're not lustful nor fearful, but you *think* about dieting every day: certainly you can't do more than that (13.10, 13.200).

Actually the morning faster is a dead-pan comedian (except when occupying a bed in the coronary care unit of a hospital, 13.323). An implacable member of the pretender clan, the morning faster displays admirable poise until devestated by negative pain (13.303; chpt. 7). Rather than revolt against their own internal tyranny, they typically shuffle time or seductions in such a way as to highlight victories and neglect defeats (tbl. 1; fig. 4). Most morning fasters, on the other hand, don't quite believe the drift of their own arguments, but derive some secondary benefit in diet talk.

It's far better to stick with the advised three regular feedings (fig. 7). Impulse hunger and consumption should be disassociated while dieting. Mere hunger of craving is not enough to justify a fattening snack, nor does the absence of hunger justify skipping a feeding, whatever the trite rationalization. Have three quite regular times each day when you plan to have nutritious consumption. Note hunger of craving dispassionately rather than be driven by it (C_6).

Understand that innumerable *diet shell games* permeate the market: cut out x so you can have y except on z if q (13.311). Don't play. Consume what you need and then fight against taking in more (chpt. 10). Reject the seductive refrain of diet fallacy.

"If her, then why not me too?"   13.305

Before your own eyes she blossoms to a level of beauty that makes you quite *envious*. From wallflower to queen of the ball because she finally got control of her long-standing weight problem (that before had made her the butt of some cruel office jokes); you can hardly believe it. Of course, you'd never admit to her how you feel about all the extra attention she now gets from the men, so you inquire through the grapevine as to how she did it.

Of course, there is some validity to judging a diet program by results. Look for the ingredients, lost FAT, adequate nutrition, and prolonged maintenance of desired weight.

The best path for you should be compatible with unique aspects of your personality, a tailored fit, because of the intimacy of controlling your naked figure. However, it is false to assume that what will work for another will necessarily work for you. *Look closely before you leap.* Diet energy is not boundless.

Abortive Onset 13.306

A massively obese woman brings her chunky, teenage daughter into the office for dieting. The mother sits with arms folded right next to her daughter. The daughter squirms a little in her chair; she stares at the "diet doctor" with cold, indifferent eyes while he begins with the fundamentals of dieting...

A derivation of familial concern, the mother fears her daughter will be FAT like herself (13.204). The mother had burned out on dieting many years ago. She justifiably believes it likely that her daughter will tread the traditional FAT path of most of the women in their family (13.203). She wrongly thinks that her powerful, unstated FAT influences could be challenged in her daughter's eyes by anything some stranger would say. Children learn more by the example of their parents than by any other mechanism (fragment 4).

The daughter has *no real chance* until she herself generates a spark of rebellion against almost certain FAT as an adult. Ideally, that critical spark will be coupled to a sound diet: not extinguished for want of sound follow-up.

Overwhelmingly, those poor souls cajoled into dieting by well-intentioned intimates will fail. Never start a diet merely because of another (13.303). The starting spark must arise from the inner chambers of your own heart and most decidedly should not be reliant upon the ambitions of another. *Perfunctory dieting is futile.*

"It's not fair!" 13.307

You gain weight eating exactly what those around you stay thin eating. There are so many delicious things you want to have. You appreciate tasty food and drink more than they do yet you also seem to get FAT just thinking about eating (13.318). You diet sincerely, but get poor results because of the "chip on your shoulder" (13.306). You may also point to some unfortunate disability that limits what exercises you can do. *Self-pity* plays a major role in your life.

You're right, it's not fair, 10,000 years ago your genetic ancestors may have survived a famine because of FAT while all their skinny neighbors in the tribe died. Fortunately, all men are not created equal. Genes get shuffled around. Sexual variety and discrimination enriches the race (chpt. 8). Great leaders tend to have good ideas and plenty of passion too.

Inequality is a universal fact. Fifty push-ups to a young man motivated to exercise by macho movie music in the morning may involve far less positive pain than thirty push-ups after a hard days work when he doesn't feel so inspired (13.317). Losing four pounds across a transition between fat zones may involve significantly more resistance than losing four pounds in a given fat zone (tbl. 1).

A three times pregnant 25 y/o will typically have much more difficulty losing weight than a never pregnant 25 y/o. The elderly with chronic disability struggle more than the healthy young—pound for pound.

Diet equality numbers are tricky (13.313). Focus exclusively on your own diary numbers. Don't think too idealistically nor logically. Follow the diet diary format like a *slave* (a most unfair state). One way or another, everyone slaves, labors with some handicap.

Cast aside your worthless resentments about having to struggle more with dieting than some contrived character. Since there's absolutely no luck in dieting, your final numbers will come out right if your attitude is positively selfish rather than indignant.

"I hate to be hungry!" & "I'm starving!" 13.308

You react to a little hunger as though the sky were falling. You start out fine for a few days on your diet until the hunger bite builds to a terrible level (fig. 10). You just know you must have more than just three small feedings to survive (fig. 7). You finally break down because this deprived state, "starvation," is evil. You have a cookie to take the edge off; then another. You're doing the right thing to quit (13.315).

Appreciate that hunger, like pain, provides useful information (chpt. 5). The type of hunger—craving or starvation—must be discriminated. Negative, positive, or even tickling pains should evoke different types of response. You know you're succeeding if you're just a little hungry in a craving sense; that means your FAT is burning ($C_§$).

Shame on you to deliberately confuse hunger and starvation. Millions of children are actually starving to death in underdeveloped nations—your unbearable minimum would be a banquet to them (tbl. 3). The United States has 5% of the world population yet consumes 25% of the goods on earth (13.307). Unfortunately, whether you clean your plate or not they'll still be starving in Africa. So you needn't feel guilty about not eating something simply because it was served to you. Your diminishing mass is FAT; theirs is muscle.

Note the distinctions between positive and negative pain also apply to hunger, a form of pain. Consume your smaller portions slowly. Develop a positive attitude about being a *little bit hungry* over a long haul (fig. 13). Believe that in the end you will be completely satisfied with far less than in the beginning (true 'less-is-more').

"I have no will power." 13.309

You *whimper* that you try "hard" but "cave in" when you get too hungry (13.308). You've concluded that it's not your fault—you simply have "no will power."

Your statement reflects the *misnomer* that will power is like blue eyes or blond hair—a genetic trait having to do with the shuffling of genetic cards. You can't help it if the ace of will power isn't in your hand (fig. 1).

Discard the false notion that you lack will power. Consider your existence in cosmic terms for a moment. Compared with the vast voids of outer space and the random scattering of universal dust that constitutes such trivialities as planets (as compared with immense star formations), your flickering life is quite miraculous.

Having demonstrated, by your being, the wonder of ongoing human existence (notwithstanding entropy), you most certainly possess the requisite power to tinker a bit with the relatively trivial issue of how much you eat.

Disbelieve the psychological fallacy that you lack the innate "no" power you demonstrated as a child when another child tried to thwart your will in play. You're not a puppet. *"Free will"* means choice about the pursuit of happiness. Your possibilities outnumber the stars.

Spinning Wheels 13.310

You frequently announce your intentions to diet. And you follow-up by regularly starting off with a variety of diet formats (fig. 2B). You do lose some weight every time, but then gain it back as well. You develop one diet misconception after another as you retain an assorted array of diet chatter notions.

Your cupboard has many diet products: lean-light-more-for-less labels (13.55). Sometimes you attend diet meetings and banter with like-minded dieters. Yet the final result of spinning your wheels *unproductively* is your net weight drifts up at the rate of physiologic fattening—as though you'd never dieted (fig. 3)! In a sense, you haven't.

Learned and unlearned diet losers have taught their FAT cells how to abort their diets (13.306). These "educated" FAT cells defend fatness by standard physiologic ploys to maintain the FAT status quo (fig. 10; 13.203). The habit of failing in a diet has both mental and physiologic etiology. Thus, it's better to not diet than diet and fail repetitively.

Language is a *tautology*, theorectically circular, no exit. The common "if no experience then no job but if no job then no experience" quandary confronts many teenage applicants trying to break into the job markets. Often some influence from a relative or friend can be applied to make an opportunity for a young person via empirical intervention (13.307).

Similarly, vicious cycles of dieting can be broken with the assistance of a suitable mentor (chpt. 12). The FAT logic that thwarts a dieter acts through a kind of evil spell (figs. 10, 12): when you diet you eat less but get hungry so you eat more. The mentor promotes probing the dark side of your being for *will to power* (13.200, 13.309); this dynamic principle can offset the circuitous reality thwarting a dieter. Skillful intervention can empirically override dietbuster mechanisms because human will can defy many ontological patterns by dint of practical imagination. "Man can not fly" was first surmounted by fantasy and latter surpassed by applied imagination—the airplane.

Turn the Master Graphs of Figure 2 upside down and you have five attempts at flying. Only ϵ breaks out of the gravitational pull of aging and associates with the other stars. The high plateaus of figures 11 and 13 represent attainment of a significantly better status quo of living in which fat cells have natural, crucial roles (chpt. 3). The merry-go-round of spinning your diet wheel in false settings can be escaped by the right path (fig. 5; chpt. 6); when the mind's eye sees the true *path* then the vicious cycle stops.

Tangential Approach 13.311

Your approach to dieting highlights so-called 'diet foods' that promise satisfaction equivalent to the "real thing." Diet dinners, deserts, and snacks that "fill you up without filling you out"—how clever. You also go to diet and exercise centers which feature fantastic machines that literally help you exercise (13.317). Your tangential approach concentrates on avoidance of hunger and exercise positive pain (13.202). You invest merely money, not your main spirit.

The best use of commercial diet productions comes at your goal weight during taper (chpt. 15). There exists a plethora of diet books to swamp the imagination with distracting calorie counting or fanciful pyrotechnics (13.15). The tangential approach typifies a *"loser."* You must approach positive pain directly because you don't want the giant holes in your diet ship that come from illusory shoring (fig. 11; 13.322). The strategy of nondeviant deviation for the sake of pleasure is a circus trick (fig. 5); the vast tides of aging or lures of cheap pleasure will not be held back by such tricks (figs. 2, 3).

The moral holes punched by "semi-cheating" via "diet ice creams" or fattening meats and additives wedged in between "diet breads" are absurdly *contradictory*. It's a short backward leap from "semi-cheating" to "cheating" and the voiding of progress made (fig. 1). Construction of a personal ethic that balances food sins and pleasures at your goal weight is a delicate juggling act not amenable to extraneous items (poem 3; 13.64). While the diet world has surrealistic color empirically, it's black and white ethically (tbl. 2).

Positive pain is good (chpt. 5). Tangentiality diminishes positive pain and is therefore bad. The immediate satisfactions of illicit pleasure should shortly yield guilt. Positive pain yields short term pleasures as well as long term dividends (chpt. 16). Most people report that they don't like the exercise session per se but that they immediately feel "good" after they do so properly. Similarly, most people report that they like sweets but that they feel no ill effects once they've escaped their daily sugar addiction; they often feel "better" about themselves. The right management of the fork eliminates that sickening feeling after over-indulging (fig. 5).

Thus the evanescent satisfactions of cheating yourself with semi-fattening food yield guilt and defeat. Many people stay quite FAT overconsuming diet products. The mild unpleasantries of ten minutes of baseline exercise give way to pride in yourself the rest of the day. You can toe the cool spring waters of life interminably or dive in heartily. You can cling to the shorelines of life and fantasize about adventure or set sail for the high seas of your own horizons (fig. 11).

Life is spectacularly short. Do you want your time to be filled with tangential compromise or unadulterated pleasures? Your naked figure may well reflect your answer.

'License to Eat' 13.312

You hear snappy music and watch those gorgeous beauties joyously frolic at the beach—everybody's drinking the same colored sugar water and eating Superburgers from the town's convenient Superking Franchise. Later that evening one of the slender, sexy models does a solo on the phone declaring a "license to eat" at Superburger because of its light-lean-less buns (excess carbohydrates) and salad bar (with oily dressing).

These *lures* of tangential attitude are designed to keep customers coming in whether in a dieting or nondieting mode (13.311); they appeal strongly to the head of a FAT, hungry body (13.55).

Yet this "license" concept has merit, just define it for yourself—three pounds below your goal weight, at the bottom of your desirable weight range: have what you want at that point. Regard commercial licenses skeptically.

Calorie Counting & Hot Numbers 13.313

You calculate your calories dutifully. You fuss over the numbers for each day and strain to maximize what you can eat legitimately, just below your imagined calorie ceiling. Your near-expert mastering of the calorie tables game guides your meticulous diet product selections (13.311). You hunt and peck (like a gambler) for ways to cheat (beat the house percentages). You can produce copious records of your dieting history with neat numbers and notations in the margins.

The actual numbers of your naked figure and weight belie all your effusive work to date (fig. 1). Instead of caressing yourself or doing some serious mirror imaging, you write abstract numbers (???). Instead of capturing a useful trace of your behavior in a diet diary, you dabble with variations of calorie counting until you tire of the tedious process, "pig out" without quantification, and simply quit for awhile (fig. 2C).

Physical and emotional fatigue is a common result of pushing calorie and weight numbers down as fast as possible. If you have 50 lbs. FAT you also have approximately 175,000 calories of excess stored energy (50 lbs x 3,500 cal/lbs). Though you feel "weak" (devoid of "energy") on and off throughout a dieting day be convinced that you have plenty energy to use (fig. 7). You should generally prefer to force your FAT cells to use old, stored energy rather than seek new, snack energy (chpt. 3).

Numbers themselves are absolutely nothing. Units such as "calories" add empirical meaning to numbers in an absolute sense. Yet dieting is relative, hence the calories/day you need to lose weight steadily and safely will be quite particular for you as you move through the different fat zones, do more exercise (tbl. 1). *Feel rather than count* your way through dieting.

The serial pages of the diet diary are units of faith in yourself, like money. Modern money essentially quantifies feelings of faith in a government. Of course, faith and trust can change. Currencies fluctuate dramatically in value relative to each other over time.

The numbers on Confederate Money meant nothing after the Civil War as the state itself was "gone with the wind." The climactic page of your diet diary has the highest value because it registers your first kinesthetic feeling that your undesirable FAT state is gone forever (fig. 13).

Many rich people demonstrate the somewhat surprising truth that surplus money doesn't translate directly into happiness. Family, love, faith, respect and other unquantifiable feelings have the greatest effect on happiness; FAT itself can register personal problems with some of these important parameters.

The cold numbers of a spiritless consumption log, recipe book, or "calorie cards" have the empty emotional meaning of banking forms; these common derivations of diet books are useful in phase III, are merely distractions in phase II (13.15).

Yet if money flows in because of your work or initiative at developing your business, then the reports do glow with a sense of personal accomplishment. Your body is also your business. You are your body, a priceless shine, worthy of restoration, a fine diet diary with an eye towards shining dividends (chpt. 16).

Stars radiate fierce energies of their reactions amongst a cold, desolate universe of space. A star dieter generates "hot numbers" that release the energy of burning FAT as well as emit rays of universal sexuality as implied by a naked figure gracefully tracking across the planet.

Premature Reward & Pay-as-you-go? 13.314

You lose an impressive amount of weight during your diet *odyssey* and indulge in a previously planned helping of your favorite treat. Or, you're a "morning faster" that regularly rewards yourself each evening (13.304, 13.52). Or, you diet during the week so you feel justified in "letting go" on weekends (13.51). You guiltlessly poke holes in your diet ship because of hazy reckoning: you've earned it (fig. 11; 13.313).

Usually the beginning dieter doesn't see the iceberg beneath the tip of a "little sin," overcalculates the rewards due, and proceeds to gain back the weight lost over time (chpt. 6; fig. 2). The mentality of a premature reward courts disaster (13.315).

Changing the FAT status quo means moving from a balanced state into the imbalanced state of dieting until a thinner, new status quo is realized; otherwise, the old state tends to reassert itself (13.203). Chapter 15 delineates a way to consolidate diet gains, cautiously reward yet maintain desired balance.

"Just a Little" Sin & Noble Cheating 13.315

You properly disregard the notion of premature reward but nobly finish leftover foods not eaten by your family (13.314).

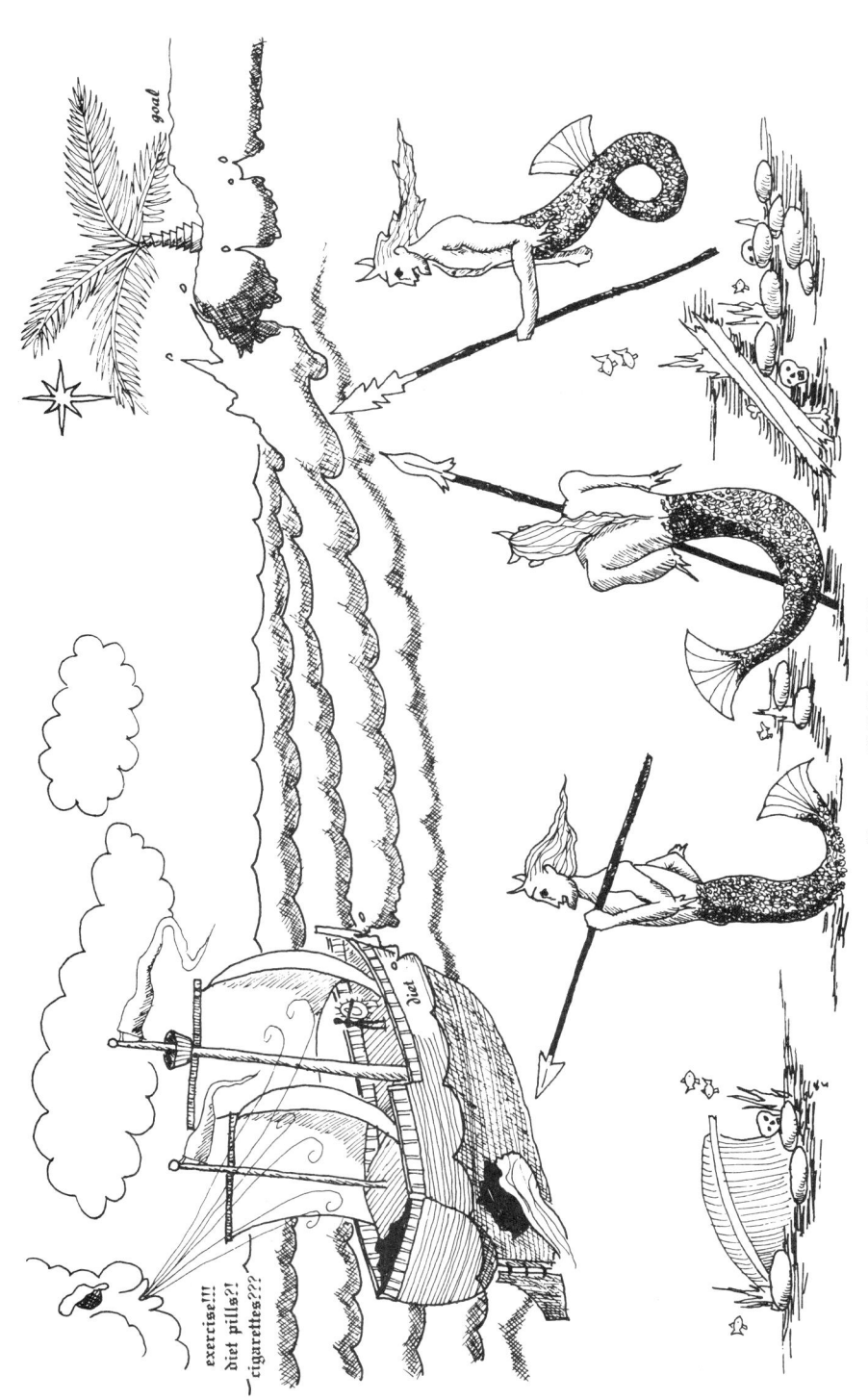

Figure 11. Hull Holes to Hell

Or, your family virtually insists that you have some of the pie you just made for them; after all, they know you want it. Though you feel guilty, you have some for their sake. They generously take full blame for your little binge because you do so much for them, not just for yourself (13.319).

Just-a-little-sin-won't-hurt mentality doesn't impress a parent of a teenager describing "just a little sex" or "just a little" pregnant. One small hole in a dike may be enough to eventually break open the dam.

Once that first unabashed sin occurs against the morality of your diet, 'serial sins' can easily ensue—"Well, I've already blown it, I might as well have some more." The prematurely deflowered virgin has more trouble saying "no" the next time. Thus dominos of sin begin to fall in rapid succession due to that casual first time. Besides ethical collapse, the inherently addictive nature of most 'poison' pleasures greatly facilitates having more (13.14; fig. 6; poems 3,4). The specious reasoning in such cases proceed with *tantalizing logic*:

> I had X.
>
> X is a sin.
>
> I am a sinner.
>
> Having more X would be more sin.
>
> Sinners will sin again unless reformed.
>
> I obviously have not reformed myself.
>
> Then I shall have more X.

Once you open negotiations with the devil don't be surprised if you get a bad deal in the end (fig. 12). Fight against even a seemingly small, noble sin because the breach in your will power may overwhelm your waning resolve to diet. The reciprocal magic of star dieting entails fostering a *discriminating attitude towards every deviation* so as not to allow the inevitable weak moments to snowball.

'Compound sin' is 'serial sin' not honestly logged in your diet diary. A golf analogy would be secretly rolling your ball over

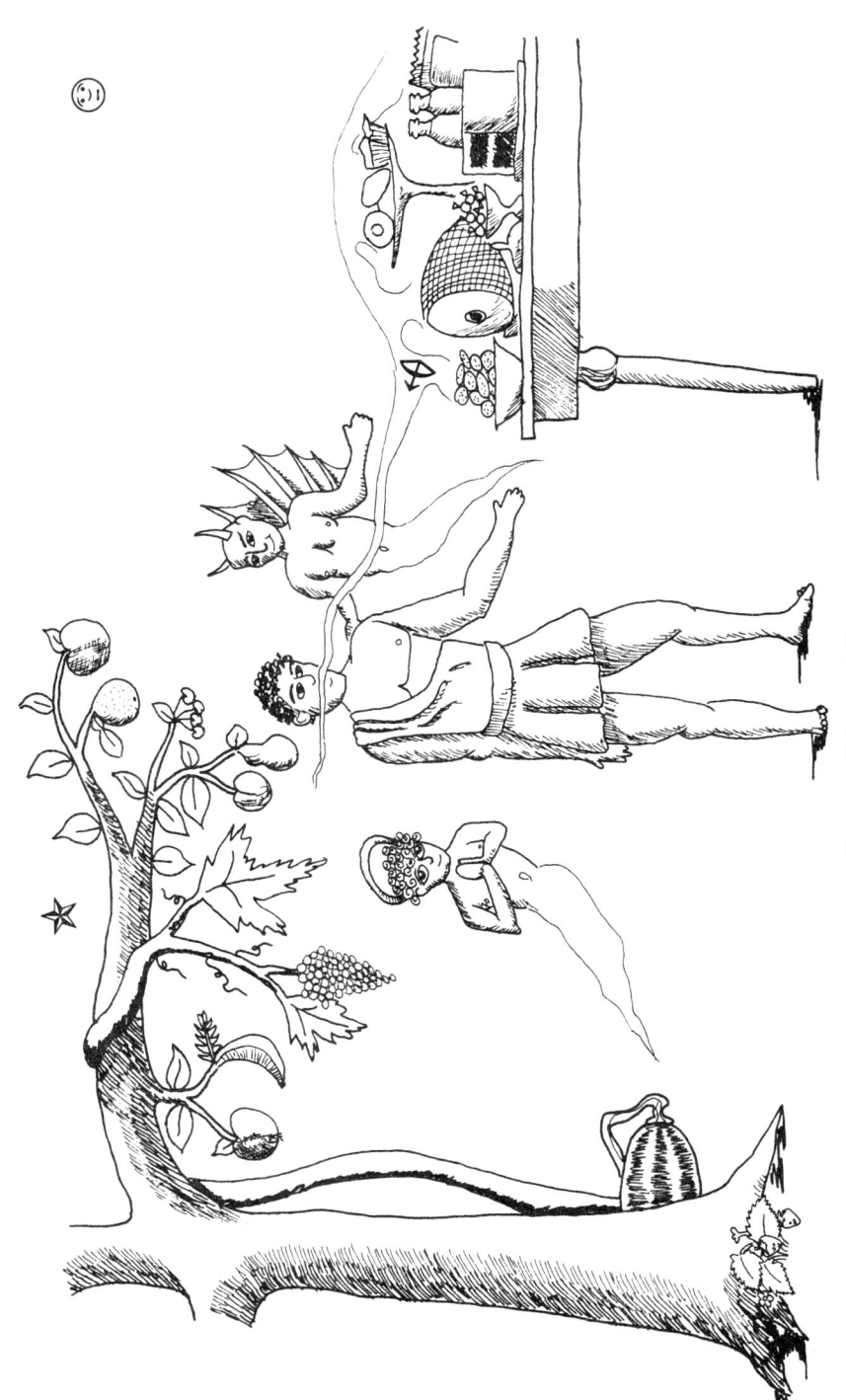

Figure 12. Victory or Defeat?

for a better lie, forgetting to record that extra stroke you took in the deep rough or that "gimme" putt you missed in the rush to the next tee. Footfaulting in tennis, "false starting" in swimming, secret signals in bridge, under reporting income to the IRS, "insider trading" on Wall Street, and a host of other "white-collar" crimes in games suggest a wanton, *self-serving mentality* (13.300).

Socrates would cringe at the perversions of logic used to rationalize unethical behavior. A simpler example of power prevarication would be pseudo-Cartesian baby logic...

I want.

Therefore, I have.

But though the scales of justice may have poor vision, the scales of weight are implacably honest. You can't con yourself. Your figure will invariably display the naked truth. You can not "fudge" to the best numbers. The diet game is more like chess—pure skill, no luck, impossible to secretly cheat. Moreover, the stakes in arbitrary sports and business games are glory and money respectively. The stakes in diet are much higher: vanity and health.

If you do sin, then write complete excuse statements in your diet diary later that day ($\mathbb{C}_2$). A contrite attitude will prepare you to do better the next time you encounter such a fork in the road (fig. 5). Ban the "forked tongue" approach because this time it's clearly in your self-interest to be totally honest. Let your own personal history of dealing with seductions guide your future improvements in performance.

Glib "No, no" & The Big "X" 13.316

You come in with a fair diet diary except for big "X's" on several days (13.51). Or, you magnanimously forgive yourself for a diet deviation by cutely inserting that's a "No, no" right next to it. You feel no guilt because life's a "crapshoot" and from time to time you just don't care one way or another. You have plenty of will power but frequently waver in resolve (rabbit complex).

Keeping an elementary diet diary runs contrary to your nature (though you did see enough sense in it to get started); so from time to time you rebel with a deliberate omission or "white collar crime" which you believe deserves a wink and a smile rather than sinner's guilt (13.315).

Sophisticated intractability characterizes this advanced form of the pretender (13.203, 13.303). Like those that would "lose and laugh" or play games exclusively "just for fun," the incorrigibles readily cast aside guilt rather than convert the force of it towards the desired state (fig. 8).

Champions are born in the labor of defeat, not its casual acceptance. While certainly it is healthy to be able to play for style or substance as well as to forget mistakes and errors in life, this "glib" attitude about dieting usually masks fear (13.200, 13.210).

As with the calorie counter, you're better off not thinking too smartly (13.313). Here the head of the FAT body gets in the way of the relationship between the hands and the FAT (fig. 1). *If* you decide you want to win after all, then stick to the diet diary format like a faithful dog (13.307). "Leap of faith" means having the courage to stop compromising yourself and "go for it!"

"I don't feel like it!" & Sour Grapes 13.317

Instead of making morning re-resolutions you've gradually been complaining more and more about the *sacrifices* of your dieting. You're losing all motivation to diet because the slow process is "getting to you." You're beginning to formulate an 'anti-resolution' of quitting indefinitely. You certainly don't feel like exercising since the work of routine chores wears you out completely, especially in light of the normal fatigue spells of lowered consumption.

The idea that you'll have to try harder as you penetrate the primary excess fat appalls you (tbl.1; 'diamond drill'). Most of the tumultuous emotions adding to the burden of the final 15 lbs. are quite unpleasant (fig. 13). It's a short step from "I don't feel like it" to sour grapes—"I never actually wanted to do this in the first place."

If people routinely felt like doing great things we'd be a super race by now. No one rushes to help the little red hen generate the wheat but everyone is ready to help eat the bread. It takes maturity to realize that only the short term agonies of production yield the high pleasures of harvest (fig. 6). Your friends will associate with your success yet don't be surprised if those same friends are not around to share the pain of production (C_5; 13.45).

It's the way you'll feel after exercising, after dieting, after the hard work that must capture your attention in those dark moments that promote quitting (chpt. 6; 13.200). Cast your eyes not to the price of capitalization but to the rewards of your desired state (13.313). Hate FAT and get past its lieutenants (fig. 8).

Yet savor the diet too, there are nice pleasures in becoming more insightful and self-satisfied on your journey. The rituals of a diet diary are designed to gradually improve habits so that feelings tend to *urge*, rather than abort, good eating and moderate exercise patterns.

Astonishing Failure   13.318

"I ought to be losing more weight, much faster, the way I've been starving myself!" Or, "What's the point of trying so hard when I lose so little at a time?" (13.307). Or, "How could I gain weight after I tried so hard all week?!"

Don't think so much. Just do your diet diary and keep going. Many of these questions have strong undercurrents of impatience, frustration, or consternation relative to imagined notions of *ought* (poem 6). Let God work on *ought*. It's often best just to write these questions in C_3 rather than overspeculate or make deductions because the host of possible answers frequently aren't worth pursuing.

'Overthought' can trigger epistemological or oncological runaways when pressed too far (13.323). The 'advanced rabbit complex' sufferers need to slow down, not move so fast: they've got to make the morning last (♬♬♬).

Consider yourself a humble sculptor working with difficult clay (your naked body): from time to time it settles peculiarly. You needn't answer every question to succeed in life...

Poem 8

Universal Education

So vast the spread of things to know
I think that I could grow and grow
At such a rate that none could go
And never sense all is that's so.

Hardcore dieters ask unfathomable questions and take the lack of answers as justification for quitting (13.303). Sophisticated diet polemics usually lead to highhanded defeat (fig. 12). Dieting is a "street thing" that withers in the hallowed halls of the academy. Hence many diet books have lackluster appeal, penned by arid authors.

An intimate knowledge of self assists the remodeling of dieting far more than extensive intellectual knowledge...

Poem 9

Elusive Nature

Can we not bind by reasoned force
Won't you be kind and not divorce
Our keen ideas from noble truth
Each model smashed by further sleuth.

Your investigations should concentrate on ways to realize the model dimensions that are within your grasp (fig. 1). Banish extraneous overthought (13.300). Seek the dreams or bright ideas that can be usefully recruited out of your dark alleys for your revolution in the streets (chpt. 10). Don't be astonished at dietbusters, expect them (figs. 8, 9, 10). Proceed up your diet road with great expectations of a climax that lasts (fig. 13).

Fatty Martyrdom 13.319

You're a good parent. You're very involved with the lives of your children. You get upset with each of their many problems. You're also deeply involved with church, social service, or hospital charity organizations. The suffering of others bothers you. So you do what you can to help.

You're anxious and involved (13.201). It's not desire nor reward but empathy that motivates you; in fact, your desires routinely take a "back seat" to what others want (13.10). Only your food desires are not sublimated for others because often it's quite convenient for you to indulge in your own delicious cooking (that you mostly do for other's sake anyway). It's just impossible for you to diet because you're always "on the go" for others—you're simply too busy to do much of anything for yourself (13.301, 13.302).

Therefore, all your FAT testifies as to your *goodness*. And your good nature goes hand in hand with your FAT. You spread joy everywhere with your fine service. Only your doctor dares to challenge the desirability of your FAT from a health perspective; your intimates know how "touchy" you are about your weight—it's in their interest not to get you mad at them (13.40). You press your doctor's staff to call in more refills because you don't want to go to the office and face his criticism of your weight. You'd rather take hypertension pills than lower your weight anyway.

So the Queen of the Subkingdom of Fatty Martyrdom is surrounded by a conspiracy of self-serving silence; it's difficult to break through the practical and psychic rationale supporting this state. The Queen must want to come out herself. Her court of intimates will resist any change in the status quo, at first (13.203, 13.46).

But the Queen does have the power to restructure her own consumption without diminishing service to others. Actually, she will be admired even more if she improves her efficiency, energy, and health as prominently illustrated through her figure (fig. 1).

Melt away the walls of your FAT prison. Cast aside the fallacious reasoning that has blocked your progress in the past. Use the *quiet desperation* you've felt all along to inspire a bold escape. Don't allow all the potential eroticism of your youth to be buried in the service of others as an adult. Make time for yourself (chpt. 9)! Your intimates benefit when you're happier.

"The pills don't work!" 13.320

You say the diet pills don't curb your appetite, the fancy machines don't improve your figure, the diet foods don't satisfy you, the doctor's prescriptions for losing weight fail. And you know because you've tried so many—found serious flaws such that it's not your fault, it's theirs. They don't work. You demand a stronger pill.

You don't work! Just getting an axe won't fell a tree—you cut it down by your *labor*. And since you labor to attack the axe, expect the tree to continue to sway in the breeze mockingly.

You say you want a "stronger pill"? Adding more sails won't help a diet ship that's taking in water (fig. 11). Adding more stimulant power won't help a locomotive that's gone off the tracks (fig. 3).

Certainly the sharpness of axes vary, but most will do if you work hard enough. Certainly seek the best diet tools you can find to trim your FAT. Adopt the attitude that you're going to get the job done regardless of caliber of assistance; even without first-class help it is certainly possible to lose weight by a *variety of methods*.

Blaming others for failure at a luckless task implies insincerity (13.303, 13.316-13.318). Apply your fiercest energies to getting the job done and not to rationalizing failure by attacking adjunctive materials.

Wrong Goal 13.321

You aim to lose 20 lbs. in one month even though you've gained those pounds over years. You want the excess weight to come off immediately because of some special event (reunion, wedding, etc.). So you begin your diet furiously and after the first week you are right on course. But the second week you hardly lose any weight.

Disgusted with your seeming lack of adequate progress you truly starve yourself for a week, lose plenty of weight, get very sick, resume eating regularly, gain back to your starting weight plus 5 lbs. (insult FAT) for all your trouble.

The 'rabbit complex' haunts many dieters with outstanding will power but totally unrealistic expectations (fig. 13). The main cure entails a steady conversion to the tortoise mode of dieting. The diet diary helps slow down those that would move too fast (13.318).

Besides tending to press for too rapid a descent, the rabbit shows a general intolerance of physiologic adjustments, transient rebounds, and voids (chpt. 14). The rabbit presumes failure: indication for *patient persistence* is the reality (13.11).

Big achievers in such social skills as "making money" wrongly think these skills should have diet skill applicability. The "leap of faith" through surrealistic diet time is done **naked** (fig. 1; chpt. 9). In this sense a diet revolution is quite egalitarian (tbl. 1).

Though the *climax* is lightning fast around your goal weight, it takes many simple small steps to set it up (fig.13). Push for too much, too fast, and you'll collapse, "choke," or "runaway" (13.200,13.323; fig. 2ծ). Appreciate the natural crescendo of dieting toward the right goal (fig. 5).

End Point Mirage 13.322

You feel terrific! You're breathing better than ever, your figure looks great, everybody says how wonderful you look now that you've lost so much weight. Your friends insist that now you have no excuse for not accepting their treats (13.45). And you yourself believe you have so much momentum that you'll just coast to your goal (13.210, 13.321). Besides, you're sick and tired of dieting.

The 'critical difference' between a winner and a champion occurs near the end (fig. 2). Attitude makes the difference. A champion hates to lose, does best under pressure, and finishes a match carefully (e.g. tennis). A winner will inexplicably change a winning strategy, choke, or simply assume he'll succeed because the numbers look favorable (13.313, 13.314).

Recognize that 'phase III' of dieting involves framing a constitution, a network of ideas promoting balance of forces within the desired weight range (chpt. 15). Redoubled effort is absolutely required near the end (tbl. 1). Many people stop short of a climax and backslide due to untoward highs or lows in feelings (fig. 13). Many new empires do not make the transition to dynasties because the *critical shift* from speculative development to conservative administration is not made.

Getting a large inheritance, winning a lottery, receiving some windfall sum of money does not convey good money management skills to the recipient. Often nightmarish scenarios follow too rapid an ascent in the worlds of money, sex, or political power (poem 4).

Cautiously execute your actions after big gains. False pride can lead to a hard fall. Learn how to *keep* what you've gained (or lost in the case of FAT). Execute the final stages carefully. Assume there's a snake in the garden (fig. 10). An end point mirage can evaporate in an instant and leave you clutching at worthless sand.

Runaways 13.323

Like tormented lost souls doomed to wander the earth forever (wearing the chains forged in life, link by link, chpt. 3), they cling fanatically to diet aberrations without end-points (13.322). Worshiping false gods supersedes good sense: alcoholism; cigarette addiction; illicit narcotic use; anorexia nervosa or bulimia; anti-exercise nihilism or exercise mania; excessive vitamin ingestion; vegetarianism or other needlessly restrictive formulae; rampant hedonism; or simply an excessive "diet" of T.V., business, gambling, sex, or sports. The anorectic eater resembles the cachexic runner, both physiologies suffer from overdoing (tbl. 1).

Between the beautiful lines, the drunken poet articulates the ultimate seduction of oblivion, loss of self, death (chpt. 5).

Behind the poignant positivism of a "get-rich-quick" entrepreneur lies a dark sense of frantic desperation, flight. Often the hedonist, who pursues certain forms of pleasure religiously, attempts to bury some form of exquisite psychic pain. An overdose of utilitarian acquiescence or pedestrian "que sera sera" prompts a great deal of diet quitting (13.47). The supreme antidieter sarcastically riddles all dieting yet most often masks exquisite sensitivity to his own FAT state: *Harken not to the Lords of Specious Reasoning (13.54).*

The "runaway" has logical arguments justifying flight from self. Perversion of desire, running from fear, or pursuing a **grand obsession** can intoxicate to the point of pseudoecstasy (fig. 6).

Star dieters search beyond reason for pleasures of enduring quality and enchanting reality (poem 14). Moreover, maximization of pleasure occurs within the framework of developed personal values that facilitate a *holistic balance* of physical and spiritual activity.

Intimates & Trigger Points 13.40

Usually intimates will interfere with your diet unwittingly, sometimes deliberately; they focus on the *flow* of a relationship rather than you yourself. It's common for people to concentrate on what you mean to them practically (do for them) rather than what you are spiritually (independent of them).

Since acquiring the diet skill is essentially an independent pursuit, the untoward distractions and diversions of relationships of service to others routinely hinder diets meant to enhance the self (poem 6).

It also follows that diet organizations built on the futile premise of dieting *with* and/or *for* others do not cultivate true dieting; *relational dieting* has a very poor track record (chpt. 2). You must diet for yourself, even if you know others will appreciate and benefit from what you accomplish (chpt. 16).

Dieting is *exquisitely vulnerable states in transition*. Intimates have a special opportunity to present fattening seductions or pique disturbing themes—personal thoughts that particularly upset you. The combination of intimate effect and nonintimate social stress presents the major external challenge to the internal process of dieting.

Real Loss 13.41

Compensation for intimate loss sometimes fuels overeating. The broken affair, smashed marriage, or forced separation create a longing that intensifies boredom and loneliness, especially in the twilight of consciousness...

Poem 10

Meeting in Dreams

I dreamt of you again last night	(☉)
As clear as now I with you then	(13.51)
And vows of love exchanged all right	(13.314)
Oh, what a way to meet again!	(13.311)
Unreal yet real I feel you call	(13.42)
And wonder why my souls still quake	(13.201)
Attuned am I your special draw	(13.13)
To nightly bliss that mocks awake.	(13.64)

Some wounds never heal and are periodically reopened. The shock of sudden widowhood, loss of child, or other major wordly loss can return with a vengeance to shatter a diet (fig. 10; 13.63). Besides the onset of winter (bad season for dieters), Christmas holiday has a particularly dark underside. Various loss injuries to the fabric of the family invariably manifest in traditional unstructured time (13.51). Somehow the anticipation, candy, and gifts do not obliterate the sense of loss. Often the post-season time lays bare the harsh reality and leads to depression. Into the gap of true unstructured time flows the unhappy memories...

Poem 11

Towards New Moon

And when I pause, my mind to clear	(13.51)
Your shadowed spirit draws so near	(13.00)
And poignant thoughts do stir my heart	(13.207)
Tis light years past our passion's part	(chpts.8,9)
Yet firmly now do want you here.	(13.15)

Resurfacing of tragedy, disease, or feud in the family ironically occurs on "special occasions." The unfairness of life often becomes a prominent motif (13.307). Deep down, the broken heart wants some kind of offsetting cure, the *pseudorespite* such as food: a pleasurable rush of warm, still fulfillment, like the secure fetal tranquility of the womb (fig. 6; chpt. 5).

Neither food nor words can actually compensate for real loss. Genuinely experience the full extent of your grief and then get on with living. Use C_3 to work out some of these feelings. Do not build upon your grief nor guilt. Pain permeates life, so should pleasure. Reach for your full extent of pleasure notwithstanding the agony of real loss.

Imagined Loss 13.42

The same compensatory mechanism applies for real and imagined loss. Basically, you *deserve* the pleasure rush of fattening foods because of your suffering; many families link expression of love to these pleasure rushes because the collective tranquility constitutes respite from the pangs of living (fig. 6; 13.41). So fear of divorcing oneself from familial traditions of security can virtually stop some dieters in high fat zones (tbl. 1). A common type of C_2 reads "I had pecan pie because my mother made it."

Frequently, a significant *kicker* of imagined loss has later been added on to the real loss. You may fantasize that the intrinsic quality of the relationship was better than the reality, e.g. that he had special qualities or loved you more than was fact. The memory of an optimist tends towards charitable distortion.

As time goes by, the imagined loss can take on more significance than the real loss itself. A diet-killing cloud of lingering despair may arise each time the dieter penetrates the tumultuous waters of primary excess weight (tbl. 1; fig. 10). Great expectations drowned in the fierce pools of life can resurface vehemently...

Poem 12

Infertility

Our unborn son, now vanquished dreams (©)
What noble form his brilliance take (chpt.6)
What art our sex could sculpture, make (chpt.8)
Once chance divine, how blackened
    seems! (13.307)

The adult seeds of expectations are sown in teenage years. Many subtle variations of imagined loss exist. Money, power, and love are involved in permutations of imagined loss. Compensatory oral addictions can arise from such notions, e.g. cigarettes (13.14).

Inability to realize career aspirations, have an orgasm, bear children, or capitalize on key opportunities can ruin a life to the point that obesity merely reflects the imagined loss. Gradual self-annihilation manifests through obesity developing at a far greater rate than can be explained by aging (fig. 3). Progressive loss of *self* then parallels the imagined loss and yet paradoxically registers as gain in body weight; if this psychic tailspin goes on too long, then the resultant crash usually destroys all chance of diet success because the germinal spirit is irrevocably cast into void (fig. 1; chpt.14).

Masochistic shadowboxing leads to no good. Discern the real loss and let the imagined loss go if it interferes with what you want now (poem 5). Use your imagination constructively. Do not organize your basic feelings around **ashes** (poem 3). Pursue the dreams that will put you into better harmony with both reality and your potentiality.

Ambush Weight 13.43

Suppose you've experienced two major waves of FAT accumulation. First, you gained to a higher plateau in the early twenties, shortly after you married and had children (fig. 3). Second, at about 30 y/o your weight rose even more dramatically to an even higher level; thereafter you just seemed to keep gaining slowly.

Further suppose that one day you decided to go back to just a few pounds above your marriage weight. Then you could expect roughly two major 'ambush weights' on the way down, because there will be a compensatory pause at those previous weights at which you had lingered for some time before major gains.

FAT cells seem to "recall" ambush weights at which they collectively established a formidable status quo (chpt. 3; 13.203). Thus an almost *compensatory void* will occur unless multiple dieting exertions have smeared the levels at which this collective effect manifests (chpt. 14).

Sometimes ambush weights have purely psychological significance. If a woman becomes markedly more attractive as she goes from being 40 to only 20 lbs. overweight the pressures of intimate jealousies may consistently manifest (13.205). Or, each time the man gets FAT down 20 lbs. his ego intervenes—he gets so cocky about his improved figure and ability to lose weight that his diet simply loses all momentum and failure ensues (13.322; figs. 2, 10).

Surmount the resistances of ambush weights by adhering to the star diet formats like a faithful dog. There's no privilege in dieting, no inner history of dieting pride to draw upon (or else you'd have no FAT now, since the diet skill need only be learned once). It's best not to improvise your way through an ambush—stick to fundamentals and don't think too much, just keep pushing down.

Spouse 13.44

If one spouse embarks on a major diet alone the other will usually show at least some signs of transient jealousy of the type shown by a husband when a pregnancy of the wife somewhat diminishes the level of her attention he receives (13.205). Sometimes diets begin because of the threat of the "other woman"—real or imagined (13.00). If the diet *spark* arises from some source of friction with the spouse, then the spouse has an enormous influence on the outcome (fig. 2).

Two types of influential indifference exist: 1) the spouse claims that weight doesn't matter and pledges enduring love irrespective of the fat level (tbl. 1), 2) the spouse acts coldly indifferent to your weight (an insult of possible sexual significance). When the crises of diet distress occur reach not for morale assistance from the indifferent spouse.

When the spouse insists on fatty red meats, excess carbohydrates, and sweet treats as usual, irrespective of your diet, then a direct challenge occurs. A tincture of separation provides the time and space for you to diet (chpt. 9); this frequently frightens away women dieters intent on preserving the marriage because any measure of separation can pry apart a fragile relationship (13.200).

Take a few moments for yourself to prepare your meals in tandem, but differently. A marriage should be able to withstand some minor deviations for the sake of bettering one party. Often young couples thinking about marriage will cling to each other publically as if to say "we're planning to stay together but aren't quite sure what we're doing, so we constantly hold hands or embrace in public to reassure ourselves." When a marriage grows stale, a similar type of *fragile thinking* prohibits any sort of growth by either party. Obviously, a successful diet could be very threatening to a feeble union.

But most couples work through the adjustments of dieting nicely. The typical spouse gives mixed signals for awhile, encourages and discourages a little from time to time, and generally does not determine resolution outcome (chpt. 2).

Once the goal weight and its attendant fanfare subsides, the couple usually establishes a modestly improved status quo (13.203). When one spouse finally succeeds at dieting don't be surprised to see some kind of self-betterment initiative by the other (chpt. 16). Great couples have dynamic *intercourse* in both physical and spiritual ways.

Friends? 13.45

True friends, like ideal mates, are difficult to find (13.44). Certainly a true friend would gladly help you through the crises of dieting or promote healthly patterns of social exercise (chpt. 5). A true friend would not tempt you with a seduction, not trigger a psychic disturbance at a vulnerable point, not be jealous of your success, not rejoice at your failure (takes indirect pressure off them).

Yet when two friends start a diet "together" predict joint failure. Like swimming across a treacherous channel shackled to one another, one friend or the other invariably pulls both to the bottom. Intimates *amplify* dietbusters through the currents of their relationship; this occurs commonly in the areas of cross encounters with seductions at the other's weak moments or cross jealousies involving themselves and quite possibly one of their spouses. Innumerable derivations of joint defeats exist.

Most significantly, two friends almost never have spontaneous diet *sparks* at the same time, so at least one is only pretending to diet (13.303). Usually, if one begins to succeed the pretender presents a seduction and subtly threatens to accuse the other of being "uppity" if that symbolic ritual of joint sin is not consummated (for the sake of the friendship).

Overall, the general *futility of leaning* on friends for diet strength is apparent. Even a mentor can only catalyze development by encouraging hand-oriented diet communication. Eschew diet talk with friends until you're done—that's just asking for a hefty dose of specious reasoning, blind advice. Dieting is not friendly; it's desolate civil war against FAT and dreaded aging (chpts. 3, 10; figs. 3, 9). Reserve comradeship for formats amenable to joint action.

Children & Dependents   13.46

At least you can expect a bit of support from spouse and friends (13.44, 13.45); this is not generally so from children. You simply can not expect them to encourage nor participate in the sacrifices you must endure to lose weight.

As primary caregiver you devote enormous amounts of energy to supporting others: cooking, cleaning, chauffeuring, clothing, tending, etc. In addition, the added services provided spouse, in-laws, or other dependents can virtually eliminate a sense of personal time (13.319; chpt. 9). The evocative ambiguity of Halloween illustrates how a "children's holiday" can present special seductions with devilish force (figs. 10, 12). Birthdays, parties, Valentines, school candy sales, and a variety of innocent formats can *ensnarl the caregiver-dieter* in defeat.

Sometimes the seductions associated with dependents are not occasioned so sweetly, particularly when the dependent is forced upon the dieter. An ill parent, dependent in-law, or handicaped child are among the types of dependents that may take vast amounts of your time and attention. Notwithstanding love or noble instincts, a feeling of excessive sacrifice of your active pleasure can be a major dietbuster.

Children and relatives are a mixed blessing of substantial personal significance. You'll be a better caregiver if you're happy with yourself. Do not feel guilty about taking some high quality time for yourself, even if you must override some minor objections due to a slight diminuation in services rendered. In a sense, dieting is *learning to parent yourself*.

It's no accident that "big stars" in the twilight of their life commonly refer to their offspring rather than their conspicuous accomplishments as being most important to them (frag. 4). Often your dependents will directly benefit from your greater vitality after you have succeeded at your diet.

'Semi-Intimate' Society   13.47

Mother-in-law feigns a big scene if you don't gratefully eat her fresh brownies like everybody else; your church friend virtually insists you try "just a little" of her fresh pie at the Sunday picnic; that backstabbing mother of one of your child's schoolmates insinuates to others how your much improved looks stem from a secret affair due to your failing marriage; the guys insist that you match them, beer for beer, while watching the "big game"; a jealous associate makes a slashing comment about "acting your age" because your more youthful appearance brings out an appealing animation in your dress and manner that subtly raises your position in office politics; these examples are dieter resistances from somewhat peripheral people.

You certainly don't want to do a "song and dance" explanation of your diet decisions every time a semi-intimate "puts you on the spot." In a sense, dieting is your admission that there's something wrong about you now which you're trying to set right. Some semi-intimates derive secondary gain by talking against people, acting against vulnerabilities in others (13.40). These "jerks" can really be upsetting.

Illiberal elements in society have a long tradition of discouraging art. Art is change in form as a function of value. **Diet art is enhancement of naked form as a function of higher value** ('star diet'). Often the main effectors of nonspecific social antagonism comes from semi-intimates: close enough to have access but far enough not to care.

As primate derivatives, we care very much about our tribal relations (chpts. 1,8,10). Society survives better, day to day, if its "dreamers" and "big talkers" have virtually no importance compared to the "workers" within the current status quo (13.203). Anarchy would ensue if everyone followed their own imagined star to excess—collective vitality would diminish. The group simply should not risk its very being on pretenders: unproven, self-oriented, revolutionary leaders (13.303). Only action (or the appearance of action) will sufficiently impress the group to the point that semi-intimates might alter beliefs. Groups like to pigeonhole people into precise "pecking orders" or expectations of behavior within a fixed hierarchy of status. Gossip, doubt, criticism, and other forms of *social friction* attend any deviant action.

Ironically, diet support groups actually hinder the individualistic leaps of faith so essential to star dieting. Paramob psychology may cajole some weight loss here and there, but enduring weight loss will elude virtually everyone embracing a tangential, social approach to a direct, private hand skill (fig. 1; 13.311).

The small slice of society which exerts semi-intimate force alters outcomes by influencing the attitude of the dieter (chpt. 2). The Arabian proverb "Never give advice in a crowd" applies both ways; it's best to avoid inaccurate diet banter as well as insufferable boasting from a would-be diet champion. Diet pianissimo.

In the beginning you're struggling to overcome the considerable 'energy of activation' (E^a) associated with moving from resolution (phase I) to war (phase II); that starting bump of figure 13 illustrates high initial resistance to this transition between phases. Each false start (resolve quickly fizzles out) psychologically raises the level of starting resistance. Burnout implies an insurmountable appearance of E^a to the chronic diet loser. In the end you're trying to overcome fear of success, false pride ambush, or an end point mirage (13.210, 13.322).

Fortunately, the pervasiveness of *indifference* provides a great deal of room to maneuver privately. Moreover, some people will offer a helping hand because they've experienced the difficulties of dieting themselves. Antagonistic semi-intimates tend to be more bluff than substance; this will be apparent if you have the courage to "call their hand."

Say "no" graciously, mention a nondiet reason obliquely, and keep control of your hands absolutely. Semi-intimate negative forces, like so many dietbusters, are only ephemeral nuisances ("ghosts") to be seen for what they are and politely disregarded. Develop an etiquette that enables you to move through semi-intimate seductions unscathed. Use some of your personal time to prepare mentally for the challenges you face repetitively. You don't have to account for your consumption decisions every time you deviate from your cultural norm; it's your private business what artistic values you embrace. *Slough off* superficial social anti-intellectualism. Once you've proven yourself by stabilizing at your goal weight, then your semi-intimates will accept your higher status routinely.

Nonintimates 13.50

Nonintimate dietbusters impersonally challenge your diet resolution over time. Active pursuit of intimate pleasures typically increases during personal time. Passive acceptance of casual pleasures occurs in business or social settings. Nonintimates have persuasive power but lack trigger-point specificity towards you (13.40). A bonafide mentor will help you acquire personalized mechanisms for dealing with recurrent, nonintimate seductions.

Your relative *passion differential* needn't change to defeat these dietbusters, just consume your pleasures more sparingly. A discriminative sense of timing is useful in optimal pursuit of pleasure as well as strategic conduct of game or war.

'Unstructured Time' 13.51

Busy time saps your energy directly or indirectly, through physical labor or emotional toil (13.301). You want to have a "good time" when you have the the opportunity (chpt. 9).

Unstructured time is work breaks, evenings, weekends, vacations, or holidays. Diets usually go **awry** during unstructured time. Drift into such time with no conscious idea how you want to manage it and you'll probably overconsume fattening food for the sake of easy pleasure (fig. 6). Specious reasoning flourishes in the evening (13.52).

Hard work sets the stage for pleasure, just as positive pain facilitates the body's quest for good health (without which pleasure is compromised, chpt. 5). Star dieting advocates an agreeable shift from some fattening pleasures to more nonfattening pleasures (chpt. 8).

Spend time with your children. Read. Write. Exercise. Play. *Develop your natural interests*. The hands of a dormant mind reach for the T.V. knob and snacks. The hands of a dynamic mind are "too busy" in constructive pursuits to develop sheepish passivity. The way hands track through personal time and space reveal more about the soul than a mere appraisal of superficial appearance.

Evening Binge 13.52

After a hard day at work you feel very hungry and tired. You can do what you want with evenings yet prefer a big meal and watching T.V. to doing anything else (13.51). Later in the evening you have a delicious snack occasioned upon a loving initiative of your appreciative spouse or the provocation of some sumptuous commercial (13.44, 13.55).

You don't think much about your diet in the evenings. When your diet resolution does cross your mind you quickly point out how you virtually "fast" in the mornings and "work hard for your money" all day long (13.304, 13.314, 13.319). You certainly don't feel like exercising by the evening and there simply isn't time during the day (13.317; chpt. 9).

You don't like being fat and dumpy. You dress cleverly, ambiguously to cover up the FAT that dominates your figure (chpt.3). Yet you "wolf down" fattening food every evening. It does bother you how *ravenous* you become in the evenings; you do o.k. during the daytime, but feel totally out of will power by night (13.309).

The general injunction for unstructured time applies to this pre-eminent example—structure it! Don't drift into the evenings without some kind of plan about activity and eating. You want to go to bed a little bit hungry, too tired to care about a fattening snack. Going to bed earlier, arising earlier yields a better caliber of personal time and promotes more creative use of it.

Exercise against the flow of fatigue and you'll fall asleep blissfully. Exercise in the morning, when you feel bright and strong, to invigorate the day. It's better to have a decent breakfast and use up that energy during the day rather than eat a big meal to be stored as FAT during the night in bed. Eat that evening meal slowly, *savor* your reasonable portions. Have no "seconds."

Do the ⁇ section of your diet diary faithfully; it's easy to "forget" your diet in the evenings (13.301). A little exercise, some reading, and a glass of warm skim milk can help you get to sleep earlier. Have fun with your children; star dieting is stylish reaffirmation of your finest childlike qualities, charm (frag. 4).

Boss & Co-workers 13.53

The boss cares about your *productivity*—not your diet. The collective psychic influences at your workplace are immense. If the boss offers you some brownies brought from his home, then how can you refuse? If your co-workers stage a spontaneous office party, then how can you not have pizza and sugar pop right along with everybody else?

The Machiavellian realities of job politics determine hiring, firing, and promotion. You are rightly concerned with not overtly trying to appear "better" than your peers; collectively, they could easily undermine your status. So you would not do *anything* to alienate your colleagues nor boss because you fear unemployment...

Poem 13

Job Hunting

Pounding turf, I seek a job
For each position ten will scramble
Each the other tries to rob
Pervading sense of heartfelt gamble
Rolling dice for just the chance
To be the one that gets to dance.

Dieting will weaken you temporarily, but attaining and holding your goal weight will ultimately strengthen your hand. Coworkers are both friends and competitors. Working buddies tend to separate emotionally if either of them precipitiously advances and leaves the other behind. The shallow support of co-workers will not extend to the depths of your diet challenge (13.47). So don't ask for help ("please don't tempt me!"). If you declare your diet and fail, then that failure will not improve your *image*. If you declare your diet and succeed, then your jealous peers may well resent the extra attention you've drawn to yourself (13.205). Diet quietly (poem 2; 13.47).

Develop an ad hoc etiquette to *inconspicuously* pursue your ideal dieting day as best you can without offending anyone (fig. 7). Of course, as your success becomes self-evident, everyone will notice—mention dieting but eschew overt declarations and long discussions about what you're doing to improve yourself. Appreciate any help you get without expecting it. Though enhanced beauty, confidence, and strength may well lead to a promotional dividend, don't suggest that this also may be in the back of your mind (chpt. 16). Try to skirt the disruptive forces associated with your work.

Getting a better job, making a sale, or simply impressing the boss is far more likely when you emit rays of self-confidence backed by a good figure. An undeniable *undercurrent* of sexual politics operates in business at both functional and advertising (image) levels. Feminists can protest interminably against sexist discrimination (which exists irrespective of contemporary laws that don't faze ancient custom), but it's a hard fact that Chance favors the prepared mind of a good-looking body (of either sex).

'Malmentor' 13.54

You send out desperate messages for help in dieting. A malmentor bounds out of the crowd and spews forth advice copiously; you act so grateful, yet you'd probably be better off saying nothing to the crowd and proceeding alone than with a *would-be* mentor out of the herd (13.47).

Or, you rush to sign up for special potions, programs, or pills graciously provided to you at your considerable expense. Or, you send for a terrific device that makes getting rid of FAT a trivial exercise (13.202). Or, you decide to "diet together" with your best friend—lean on one another for support (13.311).

The beneficent malmentor may well be a relation or friend: Beware the FAT Malmentor! (13.303). Relatives, friends, and coworkers are usually not the best mentors even if well-intentioned (13.44, 13.45, 13.53). You certainly don't want to be led by the mutually blind (chpt. 6).

Amino acid slop enriched with vitamins is so expensive and so unnecessary (tbl.2). Exercise without positive pain is positively worthless (chpt.5). The interrelational forces of diet-watch societies paradoxically promote the FAT they claim to fight by a wide variety of schemes.

You want a mentor who teaches the discrete diet hand skill (fig. 1). Obviously, the idea of becoming an expert tennis player by following the advice of a novice, drinking a potion, or buying a trick tennis racket won't work. The frivolous fluff from most movie stars on the topic of dieting rarely proves helpful.

Unlike tennis, chess, or golf (objective games of amazingly *discrete* skill levels and subjective value), the diet game has subjective operational parameters with objective value (quality of life meaning of good weight). A good mentor perceives your unique problems at ground level.

Plant your diet seed in a fertile soil. Make sure the water is pure and the sun shines knowingly (fig. 5). Choose your path according to your most discerning instincts.

Commercial Gauntlets 13.55

Football means gusto beer; birthdays license innocent cakes; wear that intoxicating perfume and he'll be obsessed with you voraciously (13.13; frag. 1). Bet you can't eat just one Wonder Chip (13.315). And who can resist the luscious smell of Celebrity Sausage on Sunday Mornings (13.51)? Tis the first cranial nerve, smell, that most pointedly integrates sex and food (chpt. 8; figs. 6, 12).

The diet road is a gauntlet (fig. 8). To get to a higher state you must get past your own peculiar set of dietbusters (figs. 9, 10). It's the private principles and not the particular passions that are the main issue.

One vivid example of commercial avenues of temptation is a *supermarket*. Note how the isles are arranged to maximize exposure of high-profit, easy to stock items that not coincidentally have high sugar, fat, salt, or carbohydrate concentrations (tbl. 2). The overwhelming offering of fattening food vs. nonfattening food gives the commericial cornucopia a decidedly anti-diet character.

You'll find the fresh produce tucked away in some corner of the store (fig. 7). Of course, not to miss out on the various diet crazes, you'll find less-lite-low-cal substitutes scattered throughout the store (13.311). But just as on T.V. or in popular living magazines you'll see one fattening advertisement after another, a brilliant cacophony of dietbusting poisons line the way to your goal weight.

Society especially won't help your diet when it threatens fast food *cash flow* (chpt. 1; 13.47). As you drive about in the city, if you get some tiny urge for fattening food you can count on some franchise being smartly placed at the next corner ready to immediately capitalize on what might well naturally pass if seduction weren't so convenient (13.53). Many streets are virtually lined with franchises delighted to *ambush* your diet for a "quick buck" (13.43).

The lucky ones have you *hooked* into the habit of going on a daily basis and don't mind offering a few token diet products to keep you coming even during your attempts at FAT elimination (13.14; fig.2). Restaurants are more interested in your pocketbook than your diet.

Run diet gauntlets courageously; avoid them altogether when you can. Take your diet diary with you as though it were *chained* to your body (chpt. 3). Read labels carefully, try to see the item in basic terms (tbl. 2; chpt. 6). Defy the siren lure of fast food signage by averting the eyes as though it doesn't exist or re-routing. Stick to your nonfattening shopping list, or buy fattening items only for your family, not yourself. When your family whirls you to that ice cream place, drive out with diet slush in your belly, a victory to record ($\mathcal{C}_1$).

Special diet friends include brown bags; plastic containers and wraps; ice buckets; fresh, mobile diet foods that you need and come to *want* regularly (13.45). A very useful term in the context of a commercial gauntlet is **"no."**

Evanescent Concentration 13.56

Long past the excitement of the brief resolution phase, you're getting bogged down in the guerrilla war of dieting. You're in the dark forest and have yet to reach the last clearing or see the final state beyond (fig. 8). You defeat conspicuous dietbusters as they arise ('advanced rabbit complex') but have great trouble tolerating the long, desolate stretches: boring.

You're tired of fruits and salads, so you decide to have a little "good food" (fig. 11). Like falling asleep at the wheel of your car on a long drive, languid deviations dangerously court a crash (13.210). You might awake in a briar patch, the diet road nowhere in sight, your weight sharply on the rise, the momentum you'd taken for granted has vanished at a critical point (fig. 2).

Golf champions fuss over every shot, even short ones that hackers take for granted, because most tournaments are essentially won by one shot. *Momentum* in tennis, football, and basketball plays a major role in outcome; often the key point can be traced back to one single shot or play that changed momentum as the champion bursts past the inspired winner whose mind had drifted off to consideration of imminent victory and the next round. Champions consistently surpass winners because of their respective attitudes towards fine details in performance plus their keener sense of preparation and execution of crucial shots.

On a long car trip, singing, chewing gum, or drinking coffee help the solitary driver stay awake (fig. 3). The imaginative use of a diet diary has similar effect (♟♟♟, ♟♟). The *master graph* constitutes a key way to visualize the internal sense of destiny, a map to guide steering through the jungle of dieting (fig. 1; tbl. 2). Brief bursts of positive pain also help one stay alert (chpt. 5).

If the original resolution is honest, then earnest follow-up, enlightened by mentor caution, will suffice to reach the high plateau (fig. 13). Once star status is attained the motivation for keeping the dream alive will simply be to hold on to the exhilarating rewards.

Miscellaneous 13.60

Eventually, human theory breaks down under the infinite weight of universal time (poem 4); e.g. the weakness of fantastico-supertechnologic-algorithmic-credentialed-ratiocinations of modern medicine comes from its "blind side" (chpt. 6). Psychiatry thrashes about in the dark looking for respect (☺). Family Practice gingerly toes the water of a futuristic paradigm of medical service (13.202). Academic Surgery and Internal Medicine proceed as though the revolution in medical business will not affect their regal state (13.203). Medical schools paradoxically proselytize the provincial anti-intellectualism and cult mechansim that typifies hysterical rationalism.

When researchers strive to develop a neurohormone effector that would inhibit craving, block positive pain (hunger of craving), they miss the point, overthink the "scientific method." Certainly medicine does good, but could do far better if blended with a keener view of the human predicament. Eventually, the modest proposal of *blissful oblivion* will be a viable alternative that modern heroes will refuse (chpts. 5, 14, 17).

Intrinsically, the dark side of medicine cleverly uses atypical-idiopathic-mixed-syndrome-type terminology to superficially label what it thinks should be locked in its parameters but behaves like an elusive ghost in the machine; fancy research should nail all such problems with a chemical cure for both the patient and the doctor's terminology: just look with more microscopic myopia.

Extrinsically, the problem of too much power relative to the ethical level of control plagues medicine, nuclear politics (the global civil war "games" between The United States and Russia, both countries founded on new philosophical movements in history), as well as the humble dieter (chpt. 10). Leaner economies are an issue. Will power is not an issue (13.309). Treaties are not the issue (chpt. 2; 13.311). The main solution consists of formulating a "new way of thinking," that manages conflicting forces within an efficacious framework (13.64).

Medicine needs more philosophy to ease vicious cycles of "tail-chasing" (13.310). Interminably, the target moves as yet another major disease surfaces to replace the vanquished one (poem 9; fig. 10). Medical science and politics have become quite reactionary to governmental spurs.

Currently, researchers look for immunological cures for cancer and acquired immunodeficiency syndrome ("AIDS"). "Magic bullets" that cure specific ills have long been the target of modern medicine; and marvelously marketed "magic" potions for obesity have great appeal. Yet much more could be done that would have behavioral impact on medical state prior to the acute need for expensive reactions, real or fake.

Diet and *attitude* impacts strongly on cancer, *morality* on AIDS. Chemotherapy has its place in agents of last resort, but how effective have medicine's agents of first resort been? A preventive medicine that takes its main cues from science will falter for lack of vision (chpt. 6; poems 7, 8, 9). The "magic of star dieting" illustrates the practical role of modern philosophy at steering science towards optimal service to mankind.

Great Projects 13.61

Dieting is easier when no other great new projects occur: starting a job, beginning college, initiating a business deal, etc. Obviously, anabolic pregnancy forces a cessation of catabolic concepts like dieting, though you should not, on the other hand, consume too wildly at any time (pica, 13.323).

If some unexpected great project intervenes in your diet, then you may keep the original spark alive by an abbreviated use of the diet diary. It's easier to resume in earnest if a trace of momentum is preserved (13.56).

A successful diet will often leverage other outcomes favorably (chpt. 16). Relax and do the best you can (poem 6). Great projects should be fun.

Near Miss 13.62

When calamity falls on an intimate, it's often not necessary to break diet stride entirely (13.15). The emotional shock waves and possible disruption of your time patterns can be mitigated by your trusty diet diary (C_d). Bad times provide a ready excuse to do what you really want: binge (chpt. 1).

Pretenders have hair-trigger diet collapse syndromes (13.303). Those afflicted with hare syndromes can lose or gain with equal rapidity occasioned upon a near miss. But a torpedo miss is a miss and technically should not sink your diet ship (fig. 11). Unfair life may well hurt one of your intimates (13.307). You'll be able to do more for them if you succeed rather than fail at your great projects (13.61). *Empathy need not extend to self-harm.*

Hit 13.63

A major injury terminates a star diet. One does not reach for the stars when thrown down to the earth violently. However, good wound healing entails accelerated *anabolism* (13.61); a special diet takes on the purpose of fostering growth and repair of damaged tissues. Some features of diet diary techniques can still be helpful.

Delicacy 13.64

The sheer power of sex must be carefully integrated into the delicate politics of marriage (13.60; chpt. 8); if this union suffers from some disequilibrium, then one or the other party frequently overeats to compensate for the anxiety or loss of pleasure that results (fig. 6; 13.00, 13.206).

Conflicts about money are usually intertwined in issues of faith. Money is faith in the state; fidelity is faith in the marriage; the diary is faith in the diet. Waning faith leads to secession, divorce, or quitting.

If no reunion occurs then the FAT divorcee will quite typically diet as a first step in rebuilding her life towards another state. Yet the diet resolution has the snowflake delicacy of a marriage vow and also requires devout dedication over a long time to *constitute* itself (chpt. 15).

The divorcee wants to establish her own sense of destiny (fig. 1). Her use of personal time could be committed to grievous overeating or to developing herself and maximizing her chances for new-found happiness (13.41). The diet becomes an important first symbol of emancipation and success at the outset. Divorced men have many of the same problems but usually regard dieting as much less important than income.

Realization of a happy reunion entails the peaceful resolution of the disparate forces typifying a civil war of marriage...

Poem 14

Towards Loving

First pristine passion led to bed
Then errors, insults, hurts exchanged
Both pointed flaws in other read
Now, over worst, towards best we range
As we persist, are we deranged
To reach and trust and love despite:
"What time or space exists for us?"

Cascading reasons reason "no"
Forget this love and let it go!
But vital instinct fires the will
Recalcitrant to deathly chill
So on towards heights, exquisite thrill
To scintillate in special flight
Somewhere in time we must unite!!

Regardless, the diet skill means the same bit of magic to either sex technically: delicate prestidigitations of handling a multitudinous array of parameters towards some special effect (political balance of powers, state of good marriage, staying in star range). There's no shame in struggling with your diet. Dietbusters are formidable foes.

Part III
FINALE

CHAPTER 14
VOID

The eye of a hurricane may pass directly over your diet boat at sea (fig. 11). Amazingly, the sun shines forth; you view a clear sky above. The green-blue waters gently lap against your hull. While off in the distance in all directions lightning crashes amongst mountainous walls of tortuous black clouds and thundering torrents of rain and hails of hell...

Or, suddenly you notice stunning silence. You're crouched in your foxhole and listen—no shooting whatsoever (chpt. 10)! You'd gotten so accustomed to at least the distant roar of cannons that the state of silence seems distinctly queer. You wonder how long this ceasefire will last; what does it mean?

Unnatural pauses at a particular *plateau* occur for several reasons along the diet path: 1) your FAT believes this diet is serious (not like most of the others) and gets quite efficient at maintaining its current size on far less blood fat globules than before (chpt. 3); 2) you've hit more resistance going into the next lower fat zone (tbl. 1); 3) your figure improves yet your weight remains the same for awhile because you're indirectly converting fat into muscle through exercise (chpt. 5; fig. 13); 4) you've hit the point at which you will go no further if you do not give up your cherished kicker (13.14); 5) you equilibrate and consolidate your weight progress so far, i.e. complex physiologic adjustments to a lowering of the FAT rheostat setting in your body (13.203, 13.43); 6) your attention is diverted to other matters yet your downward momentum offsets your letup in diet determination (13.61); 7) you've reached your goal weight and vapidly ask "Is that all there is?" (13.211).

You can stay in limbo for weeks or even months, without any further progress in your diet. Obviously, the typical reaction after several weeks of stalled weight reduction is to consider quitting. Certainly, it's important to get under sail in some positive direction before entropic currents finally take hold ("drifting" fig. 2).

If a specific problem is not found, then you must stick to fundamentals and keep trying. There's no sure way to end all types of mystic voids. Developing a *theory* of explanation, right or wrong, will commonly help you weather the storm about nothing.

CHAPTER 15

CONSTITUTIONAL CLIMAX

While her lover slept peacefully, she rose from the bed to take a bath. She smiled at her naked body in the full length mirror and saw her skin still suggested the radiant afterglow of their recent ecstasy. She bathed herself in luxurious waters. She noted with pride how good her figure felt now, after the diet. She returned to the bedroom, slipped into a transparent black negligee, and resolved never to get fat again. . .

Figure 13 shows why such constitutional resolutions as the above vignette are important. The revolutionary war phase ends as the weight wagon passes the goal weight stake. But a state without a real network of politically stable ideas to back it may soon be gone with the wind (13.64). Aging blows heavily (fig. 3).

The massive emotion wagon must also be brought up to the high plane. Overload the emotion wagon with highs or lows in feelings and the whole train can be pulled back down the mountain, irrespective of the technique used in dieting (☾; 13.207). The mocking, precarious state of getting what you want yet not having the mental fortitude to keep it can be illustrated in the quixotic vicissitudes of golf.

The exquisite "excess within control" feeling of "hitting the ball well" typifies a golf pro tournament leader: high performance with an almost magical combination of aggression and consistency. Though technical analysis of swing shows no discernable scientific difference from last week (when the "cut" was missed), now this *special feeling* catapults the pro to the top of the pack.

Occasionally, the weekend hacker will string some great shots together and earn a few pars or even a birdie. The hacker thus experiences the exhilarating notion of hitting the ball like a pro. But like the perennial diet loser, the hacker will just as suddenly get a quadruple bogey, and be jerked back to reality (fig. 2a; 13.303). Sudden confidence loss can even hurl a pro from the pinnacle to the bottom.

The delicacy of perpetuating the discrete tendency to win in "high class" games like golf parallels the difficulty of new, post revolutionary governments to consolidate victories after a class struggle for power (13.64). The new government tends to be insecure in its fledgling state. Overthought (specious reasoning) can wipe out liberal progress and hurl the government down (13.300). Nouveau riche have the same "problem" of money management—if they don't handle it right then they could fall just as fast as they rose.

If just moments before you first managed to "stay up" while executing a sharp turn on your new bicycle for the first time, then it's not wise to assume you can turn so sharply on loose gravel as well (chpt. 1). If you just learned how to walk or drive, it's not wise to imagine that you can safely walk or drive anywhere you please. A stern "no" when asked by your toddler if he can run out into the street to play should parallel your inner "no" when being seduced by treats above your 'trigger weight' (fig. 12; 13.46, 13.55). A bona fide mentor helps establish the requisite underpinnings for *staying thin* (chpt. 12).

If dieting were a matter of luck, then that luck would be effete with respect to administration of the new state (13.307). If a poor man wins a $1,000,000 lottery then the conclusion that he's lucky should not be made too hastily. Taxes on the winnings and his subsequent acquisitions will take far more than he may figure at first. Hasty purchases for himself and intimates will take a big bite. Distant relatives may come mooching around in droves.

Envious pseudofriends may chide him for not sharing his good fortune fully enough with them. Even true friends may feel alienated from him because of his wealth. Wealthy new friends may regard him distainfully as "new rich." Having quit his low-paying "blue-collar" job for which he was suited, he may find himself totally unsuited for a white collar job. "Shark"

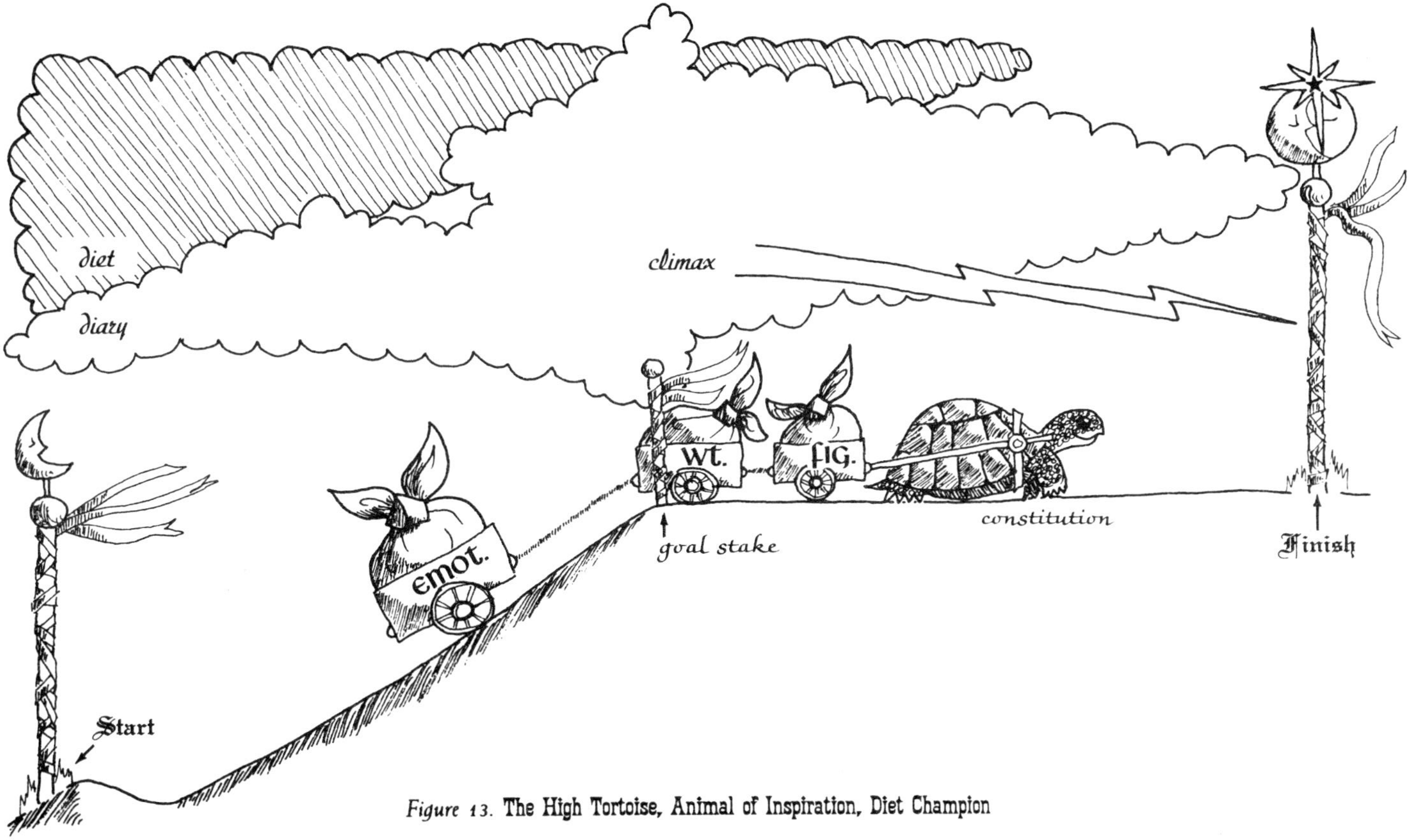

Figure 13. The High Tortoise, Animal of Inspiration, Diet Champion

investment counselors regard him as an easy "mark." Tumultuous unhappiness frequently follows such "good luck."

"Good luck" is ironically not always so different from a curse (13.210). Ideally, an unfortunate turn of events will prompt a serious quest for a "silver lining" venture that could eventually prove terrific, far better than the original state. Superstitious interpretation of real events can lead to some savage twists and turns in perspective (13.200).

Aberrant ego creates empires and/or ruin (zone "−1" or "−2" of tbl. 1). Run away from the self you presumably sought to uncover by elimination of FAT to the point of goal mass and your weight may soar again or plummet along with your psyche (fig. 2δ; 13.323). Napoleon and Hitler pressed their good luck too far, both invading Russia, biting off more than they could chew. Or, stupidly trying for an eagle and thereby ruining a good round with a resultant double bogey illustrates the seductive danger of overplaying a winning hand (opposite of choking, 13.210).

So, the *conservative skills* of managing weight at the goal level differ from the liberal mechanisms of getting there. If X equals the months spent formally dieting, then X/3 equals the approximate additional time that should be spent developing a stable constitution: **vectorial balancing** of upward forces of aging, FAT, lust, and stress against the downward forces of aesthetics, muscle, desire, and poise (13.64).

Christian ideology serves as a major reference point for the U.S. Declaration and Constitution. Similarly, the star diet applies a stable network of Christian, civilized ideas against the desultory tides of barbaric entropy (tbl. 2). An enduring state has both the backing of a family of good ideas and the flexibility to handle protean challenges (fig. 10).

The devil, aging, and unadulterated quest for selfish pleasure apply relentless pressures against a man seeking to do good. Health, family, and quality of life are major issues that interface with diet (chpt. 16). Though not as blatantly heroic as a surgeon's dramatic save or the internist's perfect selection of the right drug and dose in crisis, diet is a very powerful force in medicine (13.60). Coronary care units of hospitals are emptier

Constitutional Climax 143

more due to improvements in the national diet and exercise habits than exotic new surgical sutures for the heart or fantastic new drugs for the cardiovascular system.

Taper off diet pills in phase III (figs. 3, 11). Stop writing small details and begin to phase out your diet diary. Use conventional diet products to aid in your adjustment to your goal weight while re-expanding your scope of consumption. Diet books and fads have some interesting features that you may want to employ partially.

Celebrity-backed diet and exercise programs also add a dimension of socialization to the task of stabilizing at your goal weight. Motivational entertainment has merit in any long process so long as it doesn't interfere. You're basically looking for *gems* to grace the naked state you've fashioned.

The 'star range' flickers at goal weight plus or minus three pounds (tbl. 1). A 'trigger weight' is about four or five pounds over your goal weight. Initiate a formal "police action" when you drift up to your trigger weight to prevent the need for another diet "civil war" from a much higher weight later.

The first alert signaling trouble could be that tight fit in those fine clothes you'd bought at your goal weight. The Bolsheviks assassinated the Czar and family as if to proclaim "there's no returning to the old state" prior to the revolution. Give away or sell your FAT clothes or simply invest heavily in your wardrobe at your light weight. Irrevocable actions spur compliance to your imperial state.

Another practical way to *sense your weight* is drifting too high is through the climaxes of regular exercise. The last 5 of your routine 20 push-ups, or the final 30 sec. of your 10 min. aerobics routine will become dramatically more difficult for a relatively small weight gain. If you can only do 4 pull-ups instead of your usual 7 pull-ups, then you know there's something wrong. An extra 10 lbs. can seem like 100 lbs. in the third set of a close tennis match (13.313). Of course, if you have no regular pattern of exercise then you'll not have such perceptions and will have to rely on *elective* scale stepping to face the truth.

Whether you notice the fattening changes in the way your clothes fit, your exercise climaxes, comments from others, or simply from the scales, guilt and **savage indignation** are useful self-motivators. By investing in all those diet diary pages towards your star state, it behooves you not to get imprisoned in pedestrian FAT again (chpts. 2, 3). Many revolutions consider "freedom" a major point.

"Pay-as-you-go" thinking should dominate at your goal weight (13.314). Savor your favorite passion foods carefully, far short of addiction (13.14). Pursue other forms of pleasure vigorously (chpt. 16).

Though the time frames differ, learning to attain an orgasm parallels achieving a diet "climax" (fig. 13). Sex and diet skills overlap in artful mastery of good timing (fig. 1; chpt. 9); in this sense, star dieting is "X-rated" (fig. 6). Marriage is the political climax of romance. Like all prizes of human politics, the desired state requires courage to create and defend...

Poem 15

Warrior's Heart

With steady will you now conspire
To fuel this flame of rich desire
Keep it bright, a brilliant fire
Good signs of life that will not tire
A warrior's heart, a gun for hire
And death a distant, desert pyre.

CHAPTER 16
DIVIDENDS

Life is an adventure in time. While a successful star diet may well be the cornerstone of your heightened sense of glamor, a new era in your life, the questions naturally arise—What do you do with all that personal momentum you've developed (fig. 13; 13.211)? What is the 'delta grip' (fig. 1)?

The romantic thrust of 'star dieting' blends universal masculine and feminine impulses (fig. 6). Irritability is the touchstone of life; and organized reactivity, as traced across time and space (frg. 1), characterizes civilized will (mG; 13.309).

Once your weight has ceremoniously become a routine reality then proceed with living passionately—as though your time is indeed priceless...

Poem 16

Exotic Culmination

Some adventurers travel	(fig. 1)
Some steadfast do not	(13.203)
Some special do flourish	(fig.2e)
In the cold and the hot.	(chpt.5)
Be it mute eerie glow	(13.200)
Or thunderstorm fury	(chpt.14)
In the tropics you know	(fig.11)
One must wield in a hurry.	(fig. 9)
Spoilt fruit rots scorch fast	(13.303)
While the vibrant do thrive	(poem 6)
And the best truly last	(frag.4)
In Apollo's revive!	(poem 3)

Teachers preach faith in knowledge relatively; whereas preachers teach knowledge of faith absolutely (poems 3, 7, 8, 9). Here's a poem to a teacher in the "bible belt" that lost over 100 lbs...

Poem 17

Ode to a Once Fat Teacher

You came, your excess fat a metaphor
For poor health—your spirit caged
By pedestrian pedagogy, enraged
Your inner self ready to thrash out
Through tearful purgatory and lashing stout
Orchestrated to your feminine creed
Meaning noble hunger pain and stoic bleed
Noetic pleasure, mind to feed.

Arose thy sensuous grace
Faced darkened tender torments
Laced diary lines to trace
Your evolution, revolution embraced:
Thus we held through harsh hue weather
And after all did well together!

Many dividends can follow a successful star diet: improved looks, greater pleasure, better health, increased athleticism, enhanced self-esteem, keener intellectualism, finer use of time, leverage on other self-improvement ventures, and a more optimistic view of the future. €'s tend to develop their own subculture (fig. 2). A special dividend is teaching your children or grandchildren how to live better by your deeds rather than just words...

Fragment 4

Dedication

A good parent will personally enrich
The development of offspring by consistently
Reinforcing their finest endeavors-
Inspiring by example or involvement:
This is the lasting legacy of active loving,
Their real inheritance.

CHAPTER 17
FOLLOW-UP

No book on advanced psychomotor skills will be an entirely sufficient instructor. People need personal assistance overcoming specific problems. The slow pace of star dieting accords nicely with *correspondence* activity. You may write for an application to my correspondence program thus...

>**Star Diet Initiative**
>
>**P.A.T.H., Inc.**
>
>**P.O. Box 3203**
>
>**Bloomington, IN 47402**

"Diet" comes from the Greek "diaita," mode of living. The Philosophic Association of Therapeutic Holism, Inc. published this book as a humble contribution to the evolving spirit of mankind. The philosophic management of our burgeoning technology will determine the final path of humanity: Frankensteinian or Utopian. Moreover, the quality of inner life depends on personal philosophy.

APPENDIX I
'TERMINOLOGY' & SPECIAL SYMBOLS
'term'/symbol//specific sense//index

advanced rabbit complex
    so fast, so smartly imbued with specious reasoning & high ego that the brief bursts of dieting yield no appreciable weight loss before the "flaw" in the diet program is discovered; a/w high intelligence, success in money-making or intellectual field; pre-antidieter
      (13.318, 13.323)

ambush
    special, unexpected presentation of resistance or seduction that overwhelms the dieter
      (fig. 10)

ambush weight
    particular weight at which each diet seems to fall apart
      (13.43)

antidieter
    consummate antagonist to dieting in general, runaway specious reasoner; inspired by latent self-hate, fear, or a mixture of jealousy and nihilism
      (13.323)

antiresolution
    brief, despairing burst of self-abasement featuring specious declaration of futility, personal reason to quit
      (13.317)

black is white
    logical tenet of specious reasoning that reveals a willingness to deliberately sacrifice truth & ethics for the sake of personal gain in worldly matters: tends to sack honest completion of diet diary
      (13.300)

burned out
  capacity to "fall in love," imprint a new avocation, or generate a diet spark has been effectively vanquished with aging, "growing up;" chronic disenchantment with life
    (chpt. 1)
calorie / cal.
  unit of chemical energy in food, sometimes useful
    (see overthought)
champion
  one who maintains goal weight range doggedly; wins war
    (13.210)
choking
  paradoxical fear at brink of success that leads to failure
    (13.210)
comment 1 / C_1
  honestly logging hand motions of victory (re seductions)
    (chpts. 1, 11)
comment 2 / C_2
  honestly logging hand motions of defeat (re seductions)
    (chpts. 1, 11)
comment 3 / C_3
  sketching some emotional color of the day
    (chpt. 11)
comment 4 / C_4
  logging exercises done, positive pain endured
    (chpts. 5, 11)
comment 5 / C_5
  level of hunger at end of the day
    (tbl. 5)
compound sin
  serial sins not recorded
    (13.315)
countersentence
  mandatory, indefinite period of time (analogous to prison sentence & a/w resolution) that ☉☉ must be done faithfully until goal weight attained and stabilized
    (chpt. 2)

'Terminology' & Special Symbols 151

daily ritual / ☺♀
  logging cold, hard facts of consumption without comment
    (chpt. 11)
delta grip / δ
  realizing goals beyond phase III
    (fig. 1; 13.211; poems 14-16; fragment 4)
deviation
  consumption of unearned, "bad" items; "evil deeds" that cause upward drift on master graph
    (fig. 2; 13.316)
diamond drill
  intense, concentrated force required to lose primary FAT
    (tbl. 1)
dietbuster
  psychological agent of FAT status quo that relentlessly resists diet progress
    (chpt. 13)
diet diary / ☺☺
  dutiful data, dream diary, format of logging/organizing germane comments for self and/or mentor evaluation
    (chpts. 11, 12)
diet food
  straightforward, natural consumption as needed
    (figs. 5, 7)
diet product
  expensive, pseudogourmet items promised to ameliorate H^c
    (chpts. 5, 15; 13.311)
diet skill
  discrete, personalized ability to exist in star range
    (figs. 1, 2)
diet talk
  hallmark of malmentor ("expert"); organized noise popularized at diet fad rallies; swapping misconceptions
    (chpt. 1; 13.3)
dreams / ☺'s
  sometimes useful glimpes of primordial, dark side of soul
    (chpt. 11; 13.200)

energy of activation / E^a
  initial effort required to initiate diet
    (fig. 13 starting hump)
energy for social purpose / E^s
  episodic exercise with secondary, social gain
    (chpt. 5)
energy for work / E^w
  "exercise" for a paycheck
    (chpt. 5)
energy for yourself / E^*
  baseline, regular exercise: reasonably modulated
    (chpt. 5)
excess fat / FAT
  parasitic being ("body snatcher") that should be carefully burned off by dieting; excessive stored calorie energy
    (chpt. 3)
execute facts / $\ominus\!F$
  injunction for maintaining grip on actual consumption
    (fig. 1; chpt. 11)
fat genes
  inherited tendency to accumulate FAT on even relatively normal consumption patterns
    (chpt. 3; 13.307)
hunger hormones
  physiological cues to consume a/w H^c; typically come in tidal waves a/w specific seductions; hormones of lust
    (figs. 10, 12)
hunger of craving / H^c
  desire for deviations from right path, piqued by hormones
    (fig. 5; chpt. 5)
hunger of starving / H^s
  pathological cues to consume
    (chpts. 5, 7)
kicker
  childishly rebellious refusal to relinquish cherished deviation amongst otherwise impressive diet effort: usually #1 item of passion differential, often piggybacked
    (13.14, 13.52)

kinesthetic
  sensual appreciation of state of naked body, focus of art
    (♀♀♀)
kinesthetic gestalt
  top point of star, representing grand climax, culmination
    (see 'star diet') (13.207; fig. 13)
leap of faith
  courage to begin, make the critical difference
    (figs. 1, 2; chpt. 12; 13.307)
less is more
  tenet of diet products that promise satisfaction like the "real thing" but with far less calories; deceitful
    (13.308)
license to eat
  false or premature notion that deviations are actually just rewards (for positive pain, or cunning use of diet products, calculations)
    (13.312-13.315)
loser
  prepretender whose way of dieting consistently presages failure, invites burnout, often due to silly premise; loser of battles and war
    (contrast winner)
malmentor
  character that proselytizes specious reasoning, pills, potions, gimmicks, & devices quite oblivious to high principles; paradoxical dietbuster
    (13.54)
master graph / mG
  scientific trace of resolution outcome
    (chpt. 2)
morning ritual / ♀♀♀
  way to reinforce diet focus
    (chpt. 11)
negative addiction
  any addiction that erodes health, "bad habits"
    (13.14)

nightly ritual / ℟℟
  making relevant comments to enhance "diet consciousness"
    (chpt. 11)
omission
  deviation omitted from diet diary—"Freudian slip" or self-deceit re "facing reality" beneath resolution
    (fig. 11)
overthought
  thinking too much, doing too little
    (13.14, 13.300, 13.318, 13.60)
passion differential
  fixed, hierarchy of personal preferences for deviations; as characteristic as a fingerprint
    (13.12)
phase I
  brief inspirational burst for self-improvement culminating in genuine diet resolution
    (chpt. 2)
phase II
  long psychic struggle required to effectuate phase I
    (chpt. 10)
phase III
  crucial period of alert taper required to consolidate progress equal to one-third time of phase II
    (13.323; chpt. 15; fig. 13)
piggyback
  negative senses: deviation associated with diet product
                (e.g. jelly on diet bread)
              deviation a/w highs or lows in feeling
                (e.g. gorging on holiday or funeral
  positive sense: good health a/w vanity
              (e.g. "feeling great" a/w "looking great")
poison
  harmful or sinful assessment of deviation; desirous aversion to seductive items if above trigger weight
    (13.315)

'Terminology' & Special Symbols   155

positive addiction
  good habit (e.g. daily exercise)
    (contrast 13.14)
potion
  expensive amino acid slop or other diet product sold by questionable mentors or dubious "experts" that have no effect on acquisition of diet skill; nutritious placebo
    (chpt. 1)
pretender
  going through motions of dieting for secondary gain, but without spark
    (chpt. 1; 13.303)
principle of diminishing mass / PDM
  valid "less is more" approach; 50-75% portions eventually seem like 100% at lower FAT levels; taste & sample rather than "pig-out" when deviating and minimize hole damage
    (13.13; figs. 11, 12)
prison
  fixed web of ideas, self-spun, that manifests as obesity, addiction, depression, or consistently counterproductive hand behavior that seems impossible to change
    (13.14, 13.302)
rabbit complex
  talented, impatient, impetuous attitude in highly motivated dieter characterized by bursts of impressive weight loss followed by slip-sliding away, drifting
    (fig. 2♂; 13.11, 13.321, 13.56)
re-resolution
  repetition or refinement of resolution
    (℞)
seduction
  deviation that especially appeals to the dieter either by its nature or circumstances
    (℃₁, ℃₂)
semi-intimate
  people that have regular opportunity to make uncaring presentations of seductions, "cheap shots" at your diet
    (13.47)

serial sin
  indulging in "just a little" deviation and then justifying a subsequent deviation on the one before
    (13.315, 13.322)
sin
  deliberate deviation against ideal state a/w guilt
    (tbl. 2; poem 3; fig. 12)
spark
  dramatic, precious impulse to resolve improvement
    (chpt. 2)
specious reasoning
  high caliber diet talk a/w poor performance; manner of thought rationalizing internal failure on external factors
    (13.300)
star diet / ★
  state of education & ecstasy as integrated/consummated in mysticism: top point = kinesthetic gestalt
      upper wings = homeostatic marriage
        universal masculine & feminine
          (e.g. thrust & reception)
      lower wings = physiologic derivations
        basic sensuality & generativity
          (e.g. pleasure & children)
    (figs. 1, 6, 13; 13.10, 13.313; poems 10-16)
star range
  goal weight plus or minus three pounds
    (tbl. 1; chpt. 15)
trigger weight
  four or five pounds above goal weight
true dieting
  real spark plus genuine effort; no disingenuous features
    (chpt. 1)
void wish
  less than "death wish," but more than "apathy," deliberate shutting "off" of dynamic self & turning "on" of vicarious self habitually (e.g. T.V. "wasteland" overconsumption)
    (preface; chpts. 5, 14)

'Terminology' & Special Symbols

winner
 frequent winner of battles yet loser of war
  (compare rabbit complex, contrast champion) (fig. 2☽)
X-rated
 erotic power tapped in star diet is not suited for the immature; universal trace or sex appeal ultimately refers to the way the naked body tracks through time & space
  (preface; poems 4, 11, 14; fig. 6; fragment 1)

APPENDIX II
GENERAL REFERENCES & NOTES
source/idea/index

Adler, Mortimer
   power of philosophy & potential role in modern leadership
      (compare Einstein) (preface)

Aristotle
   cathartic value of drama, mentor confrontation of dieter on aesthetic terms, body as art, exercise as drama/time
      (chpts. 1, 5, 9, 12)

Bacon, Francis
   "knowledge itself is power" knowledge of self is will power
      (preface; 13.309)

Bentham, Jeremy
   hedonistic calculus, towards overall pleasure maximization and pain minimization
      (compare de Sade) (preface; 13.10; chpt. 5)

Bergson, Henri
   intuition and psychic time re evaluation and diet journey
      (chpts. 9, 11, 12)

Berkeley, George
   FAT prison an inescapable "reality" of bad ideas (habit)
      (contrast Santayana)

Blake, William
   general imagery, mocking medicine & scientific "progress" re fundamental reality of human predicament
      (see Swift) (figs. 1,8,9,10,11,12; poems 7,8,9; 13.60)

Bonaparte, Napoleon
   runaway ego, overcoming handicap; grand strategic blunder
      (compare Hitler) (chpts. 3, 10; 13.307, 13.318, 13.323)

General References & Notes

Bulgakov, Mikhail
  modus operandi; way of mixing medicine, religion, & politics; distortion of Christ in Holy Bible
    (compare Kierkegaard) (preface; poem 3)

Caesar, Julius
  ideal state, backed by power but gutted in ambush
    (preface; 13.43)

Carroll, Lewis
  "too busy" ("white rabbit" at outset); bunny hop desire, psychic journey
    (compare Shah, see Kafka) (13.301; 13.11; fig. 8)

Coleridge, Samuel Taylor
  an adventurer's ancient insights & marriage foundation
    (compare Melville) (poem 4)

Confucius
  beneficent mentor, applied wisdom
    (chpt. 12)

Darwin, Charles
  "natural selection" & dieter evolution, patient change
    (chpt. 8)

Descartes, Rene
  parody on "I think, therefore I am"; ghost in machine
    (preface; chpt. 3; 13.315, 13.60)

Dickens, Charles
  FAT chains forged in life, haunted souls, dietbuster
    (chpt. 3; 13.323)

Einstein, Albert
  "new way of thinking" indeed
    (preface) (13.60)

Elliot, T.S.
  wasteland of hollow values contributes to FAT State
    (preface; 13.319)

Freud, Sigmund
  "war neuroses" or ego conflicts in civil war re FAT; terrain of battle for pleasure and redemption; crusade for inner peace against main problem of age—"anxiety"
    (compare Holy Bible) (☉'ṣ; chpt. 10; figs. 6, 8-12; 13.201)

Frost, Robert
  returning to "the road not taken" & making a difference
    (fig. 5)
Gandhi, Mahatma
  self-knowledge that ultimately affords salvation
    (compare Hesse) (poems 2, 6)
Hesse, Hermann
  east-west winds along path to Om, Oz, Eden
    (fig. 8)
Hitler, Adolf
  runaway ego, blaming others, wrong goals
    (13.320; 13.321; 13.323)
Holy Bible
  as literature & a powerful mechanism for shaping behavior; constructive use of "sin" & "guilt"
    (contrast Bulgakov) (tbl. 2; poem 3; fig. 12)
Homer
  Achilles, dreams in wartime, heroic weaknesses & physical handicaps that limit exercise; diet odyssey
    (compare Freud, Nietzsche) (☺'s;chpts.5,10,13; fig. 11)
Hutchins, Robert
  'star diet' as application of liberal education, improving values as a main task in America
    (preface)
James, William
  truth filtered through tender "empathy" & tough empiricism
    (see U.S. Constitution)
Kafka, Franz
  "Country Doctor" & surrealism
    (☺'s)
Kierkegaard, Soren
  "intelligence" as enemy; the truth of Christ
    (chpt. 13; tbl. 2)
Marx, Karl
  work "alienation" & desperation ("quiet" for Thoreau) bolstering a bourgeoisie FAT State & indicating revolution
    (tbl. 1; 13.301)

General References & Notes

Melville, Herman
  spirit of adventure, getting off FAT, lazy shores of life
    (13.311; fig. 11; poem 16)
Musashi, Miyamoto
  battling many seductions simultaneously, pen & sword
    (figs. 9, 10; ☉☉; poem 15)
Mythology
  heroic ideals, supernatural imagery; Merlin & magic
    (see Nietzsche) (poem 1; chpts. 9, 12, 14)
Nietzsche, Friedrich
  Dionysus as major pleasure principle of "good times";
  nature of power; ascent from dark quagmire, godless void
    (compare Freud; see Holy Bible; contrast Hitler) (poem 1;
    figs. 1, 6; chpts. 9, 12, 14; 13.309)
Peirce, Charles
  "Fixation of Belief"; values in a universe of chance
    (preface, poem 7)
Plato
  Good; analysis of specious reasoning; "pretender"
    (tbl. 2; chpt. 13)
Puzo, Mario
  sub-cultural integrity vs. assimilation/disintegration
    (fig. 2ϵ; chpt. 16)
Roosevelt, Franklin
  fear of fear in war times (diet)
    (chpt. 10; 13.200, 13.307)
Sade, de
  potential pleasure derivations of positive pain
    (chpt. 5)
Santayana, George
  ideas as ephemeral, "sensuous and trivial"
    (compare 'diet talk'; contrast Berkeley)
Sartre, J.P.
  "No Exit" as psychological prison of FAT; leap of faith
    (compare Tillich) (fig. 1; 13.14, 13.310)
Shah, Idries
  specific experientialism & diet patient reality, quest
    (preface)

Shakespeare, William
  human nature; strange talk but 'method in madness'
    (chpt. 1)
Socrates
  diet as dialectic towards the self-good; cornerstone of "second life" (after first life of major mistake/learning)
    (compare Plato) (13.3; chpts. 16, 17)
Swift, Jonathan
  "Modest Proposal"; voyage to medical school & a hefty dose of Laputan logic; savage indignation
    (chpts. 1, 5, 15; 13.60)
Thales
  anecdote point: not blinded to practical realities by gazing at stars (thus stumbling into holes occasionally) but shrewdly aware of the ultimate power of philosophy
    (preface; chpts. 1, 15; poem 14)
Tillich, Paul
  "Courage To Be"; religious/practical affirmation of self through the star diet process
    (chapt. 5; 13.2; poems 1, 3, 5, 6; frag. 3)
U.S. Declaration & Constitution
  a stable network of ideas, linked to Holy Bible, that illustrates practical application of ethics inspiring concept of diet as enhanced productivity, leanness; "pursuit of happiness" & free will
    (tbls. 1, 2, 4, 5; chpts 5, 11; 13.309, 13.64)
Wordsworth, William
  "The World Is Too Much With Us"
    (13.201, 13.301)

ABOUT THE AUTHOR

David R. Ware was born in Indianapolis, Indiana. He received a B.A. in Philosophy and a B.S. in Chemistry from the University of South Florida in 1977. He worked as a clinical chemistry technician in a pathology laboratory before going to medical school. He graduated from the University of Miami Medical School in 1982 and was a surgical resident at Jackson Memorial Hospital, Miami, Florida. He began General Practice in Bedford, Indiana.

He's Chairman of Indiana Medical Arts Association, P.C. He has a wife and two children. His special interests include piano, tennis, swimming, golf, chess, bridge, and poetry.